Casebook of
Psychosomatic Medicine

James A. Bourgeois, O.D., M.D.
Debra Kahn, M.D.
Kemuel L. Philbrick, M.D.
John Michael Bostwick, M.D.

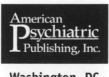

American
Psychiatric
Publishing, Inc.

Washington, DC
London, England

Purchasers of 25–99 copies of this or any other APPI title are eligible for a 20% discount; please contact APPI Customer Service at appi@psych.org or 800-368-5777. For 100 or more copies of the same title, e-mail bulksales@psych.org for a price quote.

Copyright © 2009 American Psychiatric Publishing, Inc.
ALL RIGHTS RESERVED

Manufactured in the United States of America on acid-free paper
12 11 10 09 08   5 4 3 2 1
First Edition

Typeset in Adobe Janson and ITC Officina Sans.

American Psychiatric Publishing, Inc.
1000 Wilson Boulevard
Arlington, VA 22209-3901
www.appi.org

Library of Congress Cataloging-in-Publication Data
Casebook of psychosomatic medicine / James A. Bourgeois ... [et al.]. -- 1st ed.
    p. ; cm.
  Includes bibliographical references and index.
  ISBN 978-1-58562-299-3 (alk. paper)
  1. Medicine, Psychosomatic--Case studies. 2. Psychological manifestations of general diseases--Case studies. I. Bourgeois, James.
  [DNLM: 1. Psychosomatic Medicine--methods. 2. Mental Disorders--complications. 3. Psychophysiologic Disorders. WM 90 C337 2009]
  RC49.C38 2009
  616.08--dc22

                                                              2008037970

British Library Cataloguing in Publication Data
A CIP record is available from the British Library.

*This book is dedicated to our patients
(who are often our best teachers)
and to our mentors and colleagues
in psychosomatic medicine.*

CONTENTS

CONTRIBUTORS

James A. Bourgeois, O.D., M.D.
Alan Stoudemire Professor of Psychosomatic Medicine, Department of Psychiatry and Behavioral Sciences, University of California, Davis Medical Center, Sacramento, California

Debra Kahn, M.D.
Assistant Clinical Professor, Department of Psychiatry and Behavioral Sciences, University of California, Davis Medical Center, Sacramento, California

Kemuel L. Philbrick, M.D.
Assistant Professor of Psychiatry, Mayo Medical School, College of Medicine, and Consultant in Psychiatry, Mayo Clinic, Rochester, Minnesota

John Michael Bostwick, M.D.
Associate Professor of Psychiatry, Mayo Medical School, College of Medicine, and Consultant in Psychiatry, Mayo Clinic, Rochester, Minnesota

PREFACE

The practice of medicine, especially psychosomatic medicine, is inherently reliant on the physician's ability to creatively apply skills derived from informed clinical experience to the care of individual patients. As a result, despite the enormous progress in the basic sciences, the study of the "compelling case" will continue to be a major method of clinical learning for the psychosomatic medicine psychiatrist. Indeed, appreciation of the importance of the individual patient's story, the uniqueness of experience of systemic and psychiatric illness, and the patient's characteristic responses to the challenges of illness and adaptation remain among the more important aspects of these psychiatrists' clinical skills.

This volume seeks to provide the reader with a series of explanatory and illustrative clinical vignettes that are classified according to the primary physical illness associated with various specialties. The final chapter contains several cases specific to the disruptive nature of psychosis in the general medical context; these cases do not fit "cleanly" into illness classifications. These cases are "real" in the sense that they represent the authors' own cases. Clinical and demographic details have been modified to preserve patient privacy, and in some cases composites are used in lieu of individual cases. Inclusion of relevant psychodynamic material has been preserved because this often leads to a deeper understanding of the clinical issues at hand. These cases derive from our firsthand experience in psychosomatic medicine services at tertiary-care university medical centers; in that sense, these cases may well resonate with the experiences of psychosomatic medicine psychiatrists, fellows, and residents practicing in similar institutions.

This book is both a series of compelling clinical cases that illustrate important teaching points in the practice of psychosomatic medicine and a series of concurrent case-specific reflections on the meaning of illness and suffering and the search for meaning in the context of often profoundly challenging circumstances of illness, social pressures, and other stressors. We seek to provide useful clinical instruction to the students, residents, fellows, and academic colleagues who flatter our efforts by reading and thoughtfully considering these cases. No doubt readers will have different views on the clinical histories, diagnostic impressions, and interventions we report. That is to the good; in the service of healthy debate, cases can serve as the clinical Rorschach test.

In much clinical work, there are aspects of cases about which thoughtful physicians may respectfully disagree. This may be true of psychiatry more than most other clinical specialties because of the abstract and necessarily individualized nature of the work. This difference of opinion may be greater still in psychosomatic medicine because the basic science knowledge base is still in its relative adolescence, cases inevitably resist stereotyping, and systemic comorbidity is always lurking in the background (or sometimes the foreground) to render less than full clarity to clinical impressions one may have.

We do not pretend to offer definitive management of these cases, but we do endeavor to produce thought-provoking, illustrative cases of the clinical dilemmas we all face daily on the critical interface between the psyche and the soma, both of which are threatened, variably responsive, and essentially intertwined in the rich experience of the human being and illness.

An academic note: It has been our experience that the publication of clinical case reports is an important area of psychiatric scholarship because the learning from compelling cases can be expanded to a wider audience and (it is hoped) inform incremental changes in the practice of psychosomatic medicine.

The other role of this book is to present a series of structured reminiscences of many remarkable patients. All faced various challenges, some "psychosomatic" in the classic sense that intimate psyche–soma connections were crucial to understanding their illnesses; some remarkably psychotic, with psychotic attributions to their physical illnesses; some the survivors of profound social catastrophes with concurrent need for medical hospitalization; and still others facing major systemic medical challenges with various degrees of comorbid psychopathology. The reflections on these cases at times go beyond clinical description and management and seek to illustrate the physician's own responses to psychosomatic cases and to provide material for understanding the personal aspects of these cases and their meaning.

Psychosomatic medicine is itself, paradoxically, both an ancient healing art and the newest-defined psychiatric subspecialty. It is a tremendous privilege to work in this field and to witness the valiant struggles that these patients conduct against all manner of threats, about which they have so much to teach us. We hope that the cases in this book will be of value to our colleagues who nobly serve these courageous patients.

1

CHALLENGES IN
PSYCHIATRIC ASSESSMENT

The clinical approach to patients in psychosomatic medicine often requires significant modifications to and adaptations of the clinical approach normally used in other models of psychiatry. In addition, the presentation of psychiatric illness in a medical or surgical context is often significantly different from psychiatric illness in otherwise medically stable outpatients. The cases in this chapter seek to illustrate these points.

A frequent paradox in psychosomatic medicine is that the psychiatrist in this field spends years in clinical training in communicating with patients, using varying degrees of attention to subtleties in the interpersonal field, paying attention to nuance and obliqueness in communication, and exercising measured clinical empathy—only to spend much of his or her clinical time interacting with unresponsive and/or unconscious patients. To put this another way, an important interview skill of a psychosomatic medicine psychiatrist is the ability to flexibly surmount various challenging communication barriers, often many at once.

There are relatively few psychiatry clinical models except in psychosomatic medicine in which the psychiatrist is regularly called on to evaluate unconscious, nonverbal, and/or immobile patients. A maxim to remember in dealing with cases of multiple and profound communications barriers is "the less you can interact with a patient, the more you must be a good observer." Evaluation of vital signs, level of consciousness, level of motor behavior, peripheral neurological status, skin color and texture, level of motor tone (from flaccid to rigid), and the "objective" affective state are routinely emphasized in these interviews. One may have different expectations of psychiatric status, for example, in the critically ill liver disease patient with a very sallow and jaundiced appearance than in a patient with a more "robust" physical appearance. Similarly, a patient with grossly evident right hemiplegia may be expected to be at higher risk for depression and dementia after a cerebrovascular accident than a patient with less dramatically impaired motor status. "Mapping" the patient's observed mental status onto the "matrix" of the physical condition can be a helpful exercise in understanding the patient's clinical status in an integrated way.

Other communication challenges common in the psychosomatic medicine clinical arena include

- Evaluation of patients who do not speak the physician's primary language
- Communication challenges posed by cultural practices
- Intubation and ventilation
- Delirium and dementia
- Aphasia
- Patients who are post-laryngectomy
- Patients who are many miles distant from familiar social supports
- Physical and social isolation from patients due to infection control precautions
- Facial burns or edema that mask the evaluation of affect
- Patients with limited use of upper extremities, which precludes writing
- Sensory deprivation from acute losses of vision, hearing, or other sensory systems

However, despite these communication challenges common in the practice of psychosomatic medicine, it is a truism that the patients with the most challenging communication barriers often have a great deal of psychological suffering to manage in the context of medical and surgical illness. Therefore, the often extreme efforts required of the clinician in achieving basic clinical communication are all the more necessary when one considers the degree of psychopathology in the patient waiting on the other side of the communication barrier.

Posttraumatic Stress Disorder Diagnosed Through a Telephone Interview

The patient was a 50-year-old white male refugee from the former republic of Yugoslavia. He spoke only Serbo-Croatian. He was admitted for gastrointestinal distress, anorexia, and weight loss. A psychosomatic medicine consultation was initiated for "evaluation of anxiety." The medical center where he was treated maintained a large staff of foreign language interpreters but did not have an interpreter for Serbo-Croatian. In addition, another medical center staff member with this language skill could not be found. The patient was living with relatives in the local area, but no visitors were expected for several hours. Even had family members been available to help communicate with this man, it is problematic (for issues of confidentiality and to encourage full disclosure) to use family members as "interpreters of convenience"; this is especially true of psychiatric interviewing, where extremely painful material may need to be shared.

We were able to use a telephone interpreting service, in which the interviewer composes interview questions and then, while with the patient, speaks on the telephone to an interpreter. The interpreter then translates for the patient, who has been given the telephone. The telephone then goes back to the interviewer for a translation of the patient's response. This is obviously cumbersome and significantly less efficient that typical "live, in-person" interpreter-assisted interviews, but in some circumstances it represents the only practical alternative.

By this method, we were able to piece together a tragic but remarkable story. The patient had been living in Bosnia-Herzegovina during the ethnically based civil wars in the 1990s. When his village was attacked, he and dozens of other men from his ethnic group were rounded up and shot *en masse*. He was not struck by bullets but fell under a pile of the dead and dying. To save himself, he remained motionless and silent for an extended period of time until the executioners left the scene. He then laboriously extricated himself from the pile of dead victims and fled the scene. He was eventually able to get to safety, and some time later he was able to acquire passage to the United States.

He was traumatized by daily flashbacks and frequent nightmares of the execution scene, with vivid recollections of the sounds of gunfire, the groans of other victims, and smells of death. He had a hyperactive startle reflex, chronically poor sleep, and significant survivor guilt because he was unable to reconcile why he had been able to survive when so many of his fellow villagers had not. Even after his flight to safety in the United States, his gastrointestinal symptoms appeared to have been exacerbated by anxiety associated with his posttraumatic stress disorder (PTSD). He was treated with mirtazapine for his sleep disturbance, nightmares, and anxiety. He gradually experienced improved sleep, had some diminution of his nightmares, and became less anxious on subsequent examinations.

◆ **Diagnosis: Axis I—Posttraumatic Stress Disorder, 309.81**

This tragic and poignant story had to be acquired laboriously through the telephone interpreter method described earlier. Attempts at empathy and emotional attunement were, of course, more difficult due to a relative lack of "immediacy" in interpersonal communication. Nonetheless, it was possible to connect with this man and learn his story. This case illustrates the profound challenges in communication with a patient through a cumbersome (but in this case necessary) telephone-assisted interpretation model, with the additional clinical issues of acute systemic medical illness, cultural dislocation, and social isolation with severe and chronic PTSD.

Although the specifically "psychosomatic" nature of this case is indirect, other than a logical connection between PTSD-associated chronic anxiety and gastrointestinal distress, this is the type of encounter a psychosomatic medicine psychiatrist working on an inpatient medical unit may occasionally encounter. The team was able to use this improvised communication method to evaluate the essential biopsychosocial aspects of this case. In addition, this case reminds the consulting physician to consider the tragic possibility of extreme social events such as imprisonment, torture, and attempted execution in the genesis of the suffering of some medical inpatients.

Tragically, these historical events may be more common in the lives of refugees who, by dint of their refugee status, are often less connected emotionally to caretakers. These patients may not be able to access outpatient psychotherapy services and also may be hesitant to place trust in clinical interviewers so as to disclose their stories. Psychiatrists should consider the possibility of chronic PTSD in patients presenting with chronic gastrointestinal symptoms that may be attributed to excess and unremitting anxiety. The task of the psychosomatic medicine team with such patients may also include connecting PTSD-spectrum symptoms to somatic expressions of anxiety in discussion with other physicians.

Cultural and Communication Challenges, Depression, Posttraumatic Stress Disorder, and Delirium

The patient was a 40-year-old Hispanic male without a formal psychiatric history. He spoke only Spanish, and all history was obtained through several interviews over the course of his hospitalization with the invaluable assistance of several Spanish interpreters. He was a native of an impoverished area of rural northern Mexico. He had minimal formal education, with less than a fourth grade education in Mexican schools. He had entered the United States illegally from Mexico many years previously and was a migrant farm worker. His spouse and children lived in Mexico, but because of his illegal immigrant status, he did not travel to Mexico to see them for fear of having his status discovered on reentry into the United States. He continued to support his family financially by wire transfers of money and communicated with them by mail and telephone contact.

To celebrate his 40th birthday, he and three friends (coworkers who were also illegal immigrants) went out drinking. They all became intoxicated and then drove back to their home. En route, the driver (not our patient) lost control of the car and the vehicle was involved in a single-vehicle rollover accident on a remote country road. The patient suffered a thoracic spine fracture and paraplegia. His companions, fearing discovery by the police and/or immigration authorities, and despite recognizing our patient's severe injuries, left him trapped in the destroyed car and fled the scene. He had no cellular telephone or other personal means of communication. Many hours later, he was discovered by a passerby and rescue personnel were then summoned.

The patient was immediately brought to the emergency department of a university medical center where his spinal fracture and paraplegia were evaluated. He underwent uncomplicated stabilization of his spinal fracture. Because of the extreme delay in his rescue, medical and surgical management of his spinal fracture did not improve his motor function, and he was rendered permanently paraplegic. He initially required intubation and ventilatory support. He did not experience alcohol withdrawal.

Psychosomatic medicine was consulted early postoperatively to evaluate his "depressed mood and possible PTSD." His initial evaluation was accomplished while he was intubated. Because of his intubation he was nonverbal, and all early communication was done by gestures and limited writing by the patient, which was facilitated by the interpreters. Upon examination, he was depressed, mourning his loss of motor function, fearful that he would now be unable to work (he had only been capable of performing physical labor), and missing his family in Mexico. He was angry at his friends for having abandoned him in the field while seriously injured. He was most concerned that he would be unable to provide materially for his family in Mexico and that this would be an unacceptable abdication of his role as family breadwinner. He would worry obsessively about his condition and its implications to the point where he was unable to sleep at night; when he did sleep, he was bothered by nightmares of the accident.

This case provided a significant challenge for the medical center's Spanish interpreters as well. Upon debriefing with the initial interpreter, she told us that the patient's Spanish (owing to his minimal education) was extremely limited and that she had had to significantly simplify her own use of Spanish to communicate with him. In addition, he was nearly illiterate, so that written communications (relied upon because of his initial intubation) were extremely limited, laborious, and terse. The history required slow and painstaking "assembly" over several long interviews.

He was treated with mirtazapine, which improved his sleep, decreased his nightmares, and improved his mood. Eventually, he was extubated and able to speak spontaneously, so we were able to elucidate more details of his story. Due to his illegal immigrant status and financial constraints, he was ineligible for a formal physical medicine and rehabilitation admission.

Numerous contacts with his family were attempted, primarily with an uncle who lived in a different part of California and who was able to visit occasionally. However, the patient was mostly concerned that he see his wife and/or eldest son. Because of visa problems exacerbated by the patient's illegal immigrant status, his wife was not granted a visa to visit him. Transfer to a Mexican hospital was not possible. The psychosomatic medicine team conducted several interpreter-assisted interviews of this patient with the ward social worker and (by telephone from Mexico) the patient's wife. It was striking how the patient's affect brightened substantially when he was on the telephone with his wife, only to become dysphoric again after these brief calls. An additional social intervention was active involvement by Spanish-speaking Roman Catholic hospital chaplains.

Arrangements were made several times for him to be transferred to a skilled nursing facility. Unfortunately, he suffered a downward spiral over several months of hospitalization. He developed persistent pulmonary effusions that required reintubation and chest tube placement. During these episodes, he became quite agitated and delirious; he was treated with courses of risperidone with some improvement. Evaluation of cognitive function during his delirium episodes was particularly challenging because of the baseline communication barriers of language, illiteracy, and intubation. During episodes of pulmonary compromise, he requested that care be withdrawn and that he be allowed to die. The communication barriers made it impossible to discern his full understanding of the consequences of withdrawal of care, and because of his frequent episodes of delirium, the psychosomatic medicine team decided that he lacked decisional capacity to make these withdrawal of care decisions.

After lengthy and complicated negotiations, the patient's young adult son was able to visit from Mexico and serve as surrogate decision maker. After several months of a gradual downhill course with decreasing pulmonary function with an eventual prognosis of permanent ventilator dependency, and with his son's concurrence, the care approach was changed to comfort measures only. The patient died after a 1-year hospitalization, never having seen his wife or his other children.

◆ **Diagnosis: Axis I—Major Depressive Disorder, Single Episode, Severe Without Psychotic Features, 296.23; Acute Stress Disorder, 308.3; Posttraumatic Stress Disorder, 309.81; Delirium, 293.0**

This was a profoundly sad case on several dimensions and, beyond the emotional content, a great challenge for the psychosomatic medicine clinicians. Here was a man from one culture who was trying to function in a "shadow" fashion in another, all the while motivated by the need to provide materially for his family in his native land. Indeed, he appeared to function "below the radar" like several million similar illegal immigrants, regularly wiring money back home, living simply, and maintaining a reasonable degree of economic productivity. His life profoundly changed in an instant with traumatic injury and paraplegia. His prognosis might have been enhanced if he had received timely field rescue and prompt neurosurgical care to stabilize his spinal fracture and medical treatment of his acute spinal cord injury, but as it was, his motor function never improved.

The clinical challenges in the psychosomatic medicine treatment of this patient were many, varied, and profound. First and foremost was the need to communicate only in Spanish. Fortunately, in our institution, Spanish interpreters are available readily, and we were often afforded continuity with the same interpreter for several sessions. In addition, this patient's mastery of even his mother tongue was limited, so that the interpreters had to simplify their own statements and questions to the patient. He was often intubated and nonverbal, and given his limited ability to write, communication and assessment during these frequent times was difficult. He was clearly experiencing depressed mood and acute stress disorder and later developed PTSD, so his mood and anxiety themselves compromised communication.

After it became apparent how seriously and permanently he had been injured, this man became profoundly and understandably depressed. Most of all, he longed for contact with his family whom he had for so long and at great distance (not to mention personal legal risk) so endeavored to materially support. This case dramatically illustrated the basic human need for close intimate connection and the inevitable wasting away of will and hope that develops when there are ultimately insurmountable obstacles to this life-sustaining connection.

With such a patient, the threshold for psychopharmacological intervention is low and need not require formal DSM-IV-TR (American Psychiatric Association 2000) diagnostic criteria to be met. He did improve in an observable way on mirtazapine, which we maintained throughout this case. In addition, associated with his pulmonary compromise, he experienced several episodes of delirium, the management of which had to be "woven into" the matrix of his ongoing care for depression and acute stress disorder/PTSD. While all these clinical issues were ongoing, his clinical capacity to decline aggressive and curative care needed to be determined. In view of his frequent episodes of delirium, which caused great cognitive decrements, the psychosomatic team felt he lacked the capacity for this decision.

Despite enormous efforts by the various clinical services working with this man (the clinical social services and chaplaincy were groups crucially included among these), his months of suffering and struggle ended in isolation, despair, and withdrawal. Few cases have put the psychosomatic medicine service as much in a position of confronting the basic human experience of suffering, isolation, and despair as this one.

Interpreter As Paranoid Object

When practicing psychosomatic medicine in a complex cultural environment where cultural diversity is the norm, one readily adapts to the regular use of interpreters. Often, there is a dynamic in which the interpreter also serves as a "cultural broker," helping the physician better understand the cultural experience of the patient and simultaneously helping the patient more adaptively negotiate his or her way through the physician–patient encounter. There are cases, however, where the interpreter may unwillingly become part of the patient's psychodynamics in a surprising, unpredicted, and quite counterproductive way.

> The patient was a 49-year-old single white male. He had been born in Ukraine and had immigrated to the United States while in his 40s. He had received some psychiatric care in Ukraine about which he would not elaborate. He spoke Ukrainian (primarily) and some Russian. Sacramento, California (the location of the medical center), has large populations of primary Russian and Ukrainian speakers, most of whom are recent immigrants. This patient was not working but had been taken in and supported by various members of the local Ukrainian community. He was admitted to the medical center after a motor vehicle accident in which his bicycle (his primary means of transportation) was struck by a slowly moving car. He was observed and treated for minor trauma but was noted by the surgery team to be "behaving oddly." A psychosomatic medicine consultation was requested.
>
> According to a collateral telephone contact with a family member, the patient was chronically solitary, reclusive, and "odd" in his behavior; maintained no close relationships; and was profoundly distrustful of others. He carried most of his possessions with him on his bicycle, maintained only brief periods of residence with various members of the local Ukrainian community, had never married or fathered any children, and carried several thousand dollars (presumably his life's savings) in a money belt everywhere he went.
>
> He was interviewed with the assistance of a Ukrainian-speaking interpreter. The interview revealed profound paranoia with delusions of persecution and of being followed by various threatening figures. He gave evasive answers when asked of prior psychiatric illness and treatment. He was unable to provide a coherent explanation for why he carried his possessions and money everywhere, other than to say he did not trust others. He could not provide a coherent plan for self care. His cognitive examination was unremarkable.

Midway during the interview, he was noted to be studying the identification badge of the interpreter and then began to ask questions of the interpreter directly. Precipitously, he thereafter refused to answer further questions and would not talk to either the psychosomatic medicine team or the interpreter.

Upon postinterview debriefing with the interpreter, it became clear why communication had suddenly and completely broken down. The interpreter told the psychosomatic medicine team that the patient had noticed the regional accent of the interpreter (who was a native of Russia and spoke Ukrainian as a second tongue) and then looked at the interpreter's identification badge and discerned his ethnically Russian name. The patient had then stated that he "didn't trust Russians because of what happened back home." He would not elaborate on possible personal victimization at the hands of Russians. He then refused to further communicate with the interpreter, effectively ending the interview. Because of his psychosis and poor ability to organize care for himself, in the setting of a history of likely paranoid schizophrenia, he was involuntarily committed to the county mental health facility for an inpatient psychiatric evaluation after discharge from the medical center.

◆ Diagnosis: Axis I—Schizophrenia, Paranoid Type, 295.30

This case, although a brief clinical encounter and not a difficult challenge to diagnose as a psychotic disorder, is remarkable in demonstrating how the identity of the interpreter (generally understood as a either a "neutral" figure psychodynamically or perhaps as a subtle "agent" in alliance with the patient) may, in certain cases, *increase* the amount of distress experienced by the patient. It also reminds the clinician that language mastery of the interpreter (this interpreter spoke both Russian and Ukrainian and thus was generally of great help with patients from these two ethnic groups) is not the only attribute in determining the ability of an interpreter to meaningfully assist in psychosomatic medicine interviews.

In this case, the interpreter was unwittingly a provocative stimulus for the patient, despite the relative closeness one might initially, if superficially, assume (from the perspective of a North American physician) between their ethnic identities. The historical antipathy between Ukrainian and Russian ethnic groups based on historical and contemporary European cultural events can be significant and is not resolved merely by patients' relocation to a different nation. In this sense, one could construct the patient's suspiciousness of the Russian interpreter as a somewhat culturally sanctioned response and not completely delusional per se, although the patient's larger pattern of reclusive and suspicious behavior may have made such a hostile attribution of the motives of the Russian interpreter far more likely.

Severe Burns, Visual Impairment, and Posttraumatic Stress Disorder

The patient was a 25-year-old single Middle Eastern male. He was employed at his family's small retail store, where he worked with many family members. One night, a fire broke out at the store while the patient was working alone. Fearing family financial ruin if the store was destroyed (because their insurance coverage was minimal), he attempted to extinguish the fire himself rather than escape to safety. By the time the fire department arrived to fight the fire, he had experienced severe burns to the face, trunk, abdomen, and extremities. He was admitted to the burn unit, where he was found to have severe burns over more than 65% of his total body surface area. Notably, he had severe facial burns, including damage to his eyelids. He also developed exposure keratopathy due to poor lid closure and had a prolonged period of visual impairment.

The psychosomatic medicine team was called to evaluate him for altered mental status in the burn intensive care unit. He had variable level of consciousness, visual hallucinations, and cognitive impairment. He was then diagnosed with delirium. He was treated with low-dosage risperidone and gradually recovered from his delirium.

Upon recovery from delirium, he developed vivid nightmares and flashbacks. The theme of these nightmares was always that of his being trapped in the burning store, in severe pain and severely burned, but simultaneously self-blaming for not being able to do "enough" to rescue his family's business. His family was financially devastated by the loss of their business but of course was far more affected by the severe injury to their son, their eldest child, in whom they had a great deal invested for the future. With continued treatment with risperidone and supportive psychotherapy approaches, his nightmares gradually improved significantly.

After several weeks in the burn unit with many dermatological surgeries for his burns, he experienced severe contractures and deconditioning. He was eventually transferred to the physical medicine and rehabilitation service. While he was on that service his vision gradually improved, but this was followed by an additional psychological trauma.

The first day he was able to see clearly enough, he was given a mirror to look at himself for the first time since his admission. He immediately recoiled in horror when he saw the residual appearance of his facial burns. Ironically and tragically, a recent formal portrait of himself was on his nightstand. He had been a strikingly handsome young man, with strong, dark features, thick black hair, and large, warm, brown eyes. He now had severe facial scarring, abnormal eyelid apposition, and no hair. Indeed, he looked like an old and wizened man. In addition to all his other suffering, he now had to confront concretely his loss of appearance, an appearance that had likely been a source of great pride and much admiration for him.

◆ **Diagnosis: Axis I—Delirium 293.0; Posttraumatic Stress Disorder, 309.81**

This case tragically illustrates several points. Patients will often not act in their own obvious self-interest and may expose themselves to significant injuries when social and economic realities intrude. This man would probably have been able to escape the fire largely unharmed had he not felt a sense of obligation to stay and fight the fire that threatened his family's business. As the oldest son, did he feel a particularly strong need to be "heroic" and "valiant" in saving the family business? Did he fear that had he escaped and not attempted to save the family business he would have experienced some nonspecific recrimination at the hands of his family? Could he even have thought this through at the time (he later had little memory of his motivation at the time of the fire)?

Once admitted to the burn unit, he had an episode of delirium, a common problem in burn patients, for which he was treated and from which he recovered. Upon recovery, he then experienced nightmares and flashbacks of the fire consistent with PTSD. Again, with treatment, this gradually improved. Interviewing this man was particularly challenging. When initially seen, he was intubated, limiting clinical assessment. Because of burns to his hands, he could not initially hold a pen to write to the interviewers. His visual impairment had left him unable to read as well. These alone produced significant communications barriers in assessment. In addition, his severe facial burns gave him an appearance of blunted affect.

This case reminds one of how it is easy to take for granted the usual methods of human communication, and how when many of these are unavailable (no speech due to intubation, no writing due to extremity burns, minimal eye contact, and inability to read due to corneal and eyelid injury; severe limitations in the clinician's ability to "read" the patient's affect due to facial burns), there is a great sense of distance and an inability to understand the patient's internal experience. Imagine how isolated it must feel to be the patient in such a circumstance; first confused and delirious, then having PTSD symptoms due to the accident and injuries, then finally experiencing fear and despair when able to look at oneself in the mirror and see how the world will hereafter see you. The image of the severely injured, contracted, burned, and disfigured patient in the hospital bed beside the handsome, dashing formal portrait of his "former self" was one of the most touchingly ironic pairings one would expect to see.

Cognitive Impairment and Bedside Cognitive Testing

An especially frequent communication barrier in psychosomatic medicine that is much less frequent in many other areas of clinical psychiatry is work with cognitively impaired patients. One is often graphically reminded of the aphorism that in psychiatry, an important aspect of the clinical work is that the physician must communicate directly with the diseased organ, which is expected to somehow describe its own suffering. It is easy to forget for a moment how much we value our cognition in our interpersonal encounters. When communication is necessary with cognitively impaired patients, however, much cognitively based social reciprocity is lost.

The cognitively impaired patient can be quite difficult to interview in the "usual" way. Often, in the case of suspected impairment, it is a useful clinical approach to assess the patient's function with formal cognitive assessment relatively early in the interview. This accomplishes a number of goals. First, it establishes the patient's cognitive status early in the interview. If the patient is severely impaired, one would be clearly remiss in subsequently expecting the patient to accurately recall important aspects of his or her medical/surgical illness and hospitalization. Demonstrated cognitive impairment early in the clinical interview helps to guide the structure of further clinical questions. One would not ask elaborate and/or abstract questions of a patently cognitively impaired patient with any reasonable expectation of accurate answers. In addition, cognitively impaired patients frequently have impaired attention that is difficult to sustain, so formal cognitive testing should be done when the patient is at his or her relative "best."

Psychosomatic medicine clinical examination at the bedside involves assessment of several domains of mental function. Formal cognitive testing includes standardized instruments such as the Mini-Mental State Examination (MMSE; Folstein et al. 1975). In view of the limitations of the MMSE for assessment of frontal lobe function, psychiatrists routinely supplement it with other instruments to assess frontal lobe function. One of these frontal lobe function tests is a category generation test called the "animals test."

The method is simple: The patient is told "Now I would like you to name as many animals as possible until I ask you to stop." The examiner then measures 1 minute. Twelve animals in 1 minute is considered a clinically useful cutoff. In addition to the 12 responses in 1 minute, the cognitively intact patient will use a logical search strategy, such as initially naming household pets, then changing categories to farm animals, and then to wild animals. Although this is an easy task for cognitively intact patients, cognitively impaired patients often have a great deal of difficulty with it. The following are remarkable examples of responses to this test.

"Multiple Cats"

A 65-year-old man with dementia (he had a mildly decreased MMSE score of 23), narcissistic personality disorder, and alcohol dependence had had numerous difficulties in self care, and structured placement was being considered. His response to the "animals test" was thus: "Well, you got your big cats, you got yellow cats, little cats, black cats, kitty cats, I had a cat once, let me tell you about him!" (Wherein he then abandoned the test to tell us an anecdote about this particular cat). This was scored as "1." Notable was his perseveration (repeating "cat" several times), his way of modifying the adjective as though that meant another item in the required set, and his tangentiality in becoming distracted from the task by telling a story about a cat. Interestingly, the profoundly abnormal "animals test" performance actually correlated quite well with his inability at self care and decision making—much better than did his mildly impaired MMSE score. He was subsequently discharged to a structured placement.

Switching Set

The neuropsychological term "switching set" refers to the ability to change from one topic to another in response to appropriate environmental cues. Indeed, the "multiple cats" patient just described was unable to switch set from "cat" to another item. Another dementia patient had the following responses: "Cat, dog, cow, horse, fish, fish... (a few seconds of pause), fish is good with lemon, lemon, strawberry, cherry, apple...." We interpreted this as "spontaneous tangentiality." The "fish" and "lemon" are related as a common diet combination item; once he said "lemon," he then "switched set" and named fruits, never returning to the category of animals.

> A patient with a long history of profound alcohol dependence ("two 12-packs of beer a day") presented with confusion and agitation. He scored only a 10 on his MMSE and had long latency in responses, appearing to "rehearse" his often grossly inaccurate answers (e.g., the current year as "1896" and being unable to name any U.S. presidents). On the categories test, in 1 minute he could only say "boat, blue, capper, cat."

Impersistence

Many dementia patients show the ability to attend to brief cognitive tasks (e.g., the individual components of the MMSE) but fail dramatically in the requirement of the 1 minute of effort of the "animals test."

> This patient was in the early stages of Alzheimer's disease with a mildly decreased MMSE score (22) and notable apathy. His response to the "animals test" was "Dog, cat, mouse, (pause) I can't do any more." This impersistence on this task may also be seen with depressed patients.

Item Confusion

We have had several dementia or delirium patients who show their confusion and/or poor judgment quite eloquently on the "animals test" by the items chosen within the category of "animals":

"A beef."
"Is beef an animal?"
"Cantaloupe."
"Mickey, Donald, and Goofy."
"Unicorn."
"Dragon."
"Plants."
"Giant."

Repetition

We have had several dementia or delirium patients who will perseverate by returning to previously mentioned items, such as "dog, cat, mouse, horse, cow, monkey, dog, cat." They may or may not eventually name 12 or more different animals, but the repetition should be noted even if they eventually name the requisite number of different animals.

"Mr. 5150" or the Extreme-Appearance Patient

Clinical assessment in psychosomatic medicine notably also includes basic physical and behavioral observation. One is reminded that communication is a multifaceted phenomenon, because observation of the patient is itself a form of communication. Patients who electively adopt an extreme appearance (e.g., tattoos, body piercings) may be the source of significant countertransference responses that may themselves generate the need for a consultation, even if the patients' manifest behavior is otherwise not disruptive. As is illustrated in this case, communication often follows simple observation as much as it follows conversation.

> The patient was a 22-year-old single white male who was admitted to the burn service with burns suffered in a fire. The burn resident hurriedly called for a psychosomatic medicine consult, pleading that "he's really crazy." The team asked if the patient was agitated, suicidal, or incoherent, and was told, "no, he's just crazy…you'll see when you meet him." Obviously intrigued by this introduction (if also a bit jaded, because psychiatric impairment is commonly exaggerated by referring services so as to obtain a consult), the team responded promptly.
> The team entered the patient's room to encounter a slightly built young man with a shaved head. He was alert and cooperative and did

not resist the interview. He was asked if he knew that the psychoso-matic medicine team had been consulted, to which he replied "I fig-ured they would call you. I just want you to know, a lot of people think I am crazy!" He denied history of psychosis, depression, sui-cidality, homicidality, or psychotic hospitalization except that "I only see things when I take methamphetamine." He then said "Check this out!" and turned his head.

There, in large print covering much of the left side of his (shaved) head, was a tattoo of the number "5150." 5150 is the section of the California Welfare and Institutions Code pertaining to involuntary commitment of the mentally ill. In California, the number "5150" has entered the local psychiatric (and even local cultural) parlance on several levels. As a transitive verb, it is used by psychiatry resi-dents to describe the act of initiating a civil commitment (e.g., "I 5150'd Mr. Jones to the psychiatric facility last night"). In addition, lay culture in California also uses the term "5150" as a generic term for nonconformity and rebelliousness. This man could not explain his reasoning for getting this tattoo beyond the desire to impress others and for "shock value." Indeed, what else could be the moti-vation for getting this particular tattoo? In this regard, it was quite effective. With some apparent pride at impressing a consultation team, he said "You look like you've never seen a guy with a 5150 on his head before!"

He remained in stable condition without acute psychiatric symp-toms for the balance of his hospitalization. He required neither psy-chotropic medications nor transfer to a psychiatric hospital when he recovered from his burns. He had no amphetamine-related with-drawal symptoms during his hospitalization.

♦ **Diagnosis: Axis I—Amphetamine Abuse, 305.70, Rule Out Dependence; Axis II—Narcissistic and Borderline Traits, Rule Out Personality Disorder Not Otherwise Specified**

Beyond his substance use, Cluster B spectrum primitive character style, and behavioral impulsivity, this man was not otherwise men-tally ill. No doubt the impulse to get a "5150" tattooed on one's head (not to mention actually having it placed) is an unusual one and serves, at the very least, as a marker for greater impulsivity. His wish for attention was indeed promptly granted by the psychosomatic medicine consultation, although the referring surgery team contin-ued to have countertransference issues with this man. He in fact did NOT receive a "5150" commitment (because he was not acutely suicidal, homicidal, or unable to provide for his own basic needs) to "match" his tattoo.

References

American Psychiatric Association: Diagnostic and Statistical Manual of Mental Disorders, 4th Edition, Text Revision. Washington, DC, American Psychiatric Association, 2000

Folstein MF, Folstein SE, McHugh PR: "Mini-Mental State": a practical method for grading the cognitive state of patients for the clinician. J Psychiatr Res 12:189–198, 1975

2

ACUTE MENTAL STATUS CHANGES/DELIRIUM

"**A**cute mental status changes" is a common reason for consultation by the psychosomatic medicine psychiatrist. A general approach to delirium workup is needed, because delirium may occur in conditions affecting many different organ systems. In addition, the conditions of neuroleptic malignant syndrome (NMS) and serotonin syndrome may need to be considered in the differential diagnosis of the delirium patient.

The general approach of the psychosomatic medicine service to all cases of delirium is to identify the underlying causes and treat the symptoms of delirium while the responsible pathologies are being addressed. As defined by DSM-IV-TR (American Psychiatric Association 2000, p. 143), delirium is characterized by:

Disturbance of consciousness (i.e., reduced clarity of awareness of the environment) with reduced ability to focus, sustain, or shift attention.

A. A change in cognition (such as memory deficit, disorientation, language disturbance) or the development of a perceptual disturbance that is not better accounted for by a preexisting, established, or evolving dementia.
B. The disturbance develops over a short period of time (usually hours to days) and tends to fluctuate during the course of the day.
C. There is evidence from the history, physical examination, or laboratory findings that the disturbance is caused by the direct physiological consequences of a general medical condition.

Each delirium patient will have a different balance of contributing factors, but the underlying principles of diagnosis, evaluation, and treatment of delirium can be generalized across a broad range of presentations and underlying pathologies. The evaluation of delirium must primarily include an investigation of the most common causes, which include fluid and electrolyte disturbances, infections, drug toxicity and withdrawal (including medications), metabolic disorders, and low perfusion states.

Although the treatment of identified disturbances in these listed categories is essential, using psychotropic medication to treat delirium is somewhat more controversial. Small studies have found risperidone, olanzapine, and haloperidol useful in treating delirium, but objective data are limited (Lonergan et al. 2007). Other medications, such as donepezil, have been found useful for delirium in the case report literature (Slatkin and Rhiner 2004; Slatkin et al. 2001). The mechanism by which these various medications work is likely related to a correction of neurotransmitter imbalances common to delirium, although this has not been fully elucidated.

Blindness and Visual Hallucinations

Sensory deprivation may be a contributing factor to delirium. Whether sensory deprivation per se precipitates delirium is controversial; however, it is clear from clinical experience that sensory deprivation (often in the form of inadequate vision correction and/or inadequately treated hearing impairment) may add to confusion experienced by a delirious patient. We managed a tragic case in which acute onset of bilateral blindness was associated with visual hallucinations, perhaps due to acute sensory impairment.

> The patient was a 45-year-old white male with a long history of depression and alcoholism. He had had an exacerbation of his alcoholism and worsening depression for which he did not receive treatment. His depression progressed to include acute suicidality. While intoxicated, he shot himself in the head, transecting both optic nerves in the process. Remarkably, he did not suffer significant cortical damage. He was seen in consultation in the intensive care unit after initial stabilization of his injuries.
>
> He spontaneously connected his depression and alcoholism in the genesis of his tragic injury by saying "the depression made me

load the gun; the alcohol made me pull the trigger." He felt overwhelming regret over having blinded himself and was, understandably, significantly more depressed now. His family had rallied to his side, and he was able to express that he now wished to live to "be there" for his family members. With active surveillance, he did not experience symptoms of alcohol withdrawal.

After several days in the hospital, he began to report visual hallucinations. These consisted of both formed and unformed images and frequently were the images of people he knew. When confronted, he was always able to recall that he had blinded himself; thus, he was not "psychotically" denying the tragic fact of his blindness. Rather, he was experiencing visual sensations without receiving visual information from the environment. We explained to him that our understanding of his condition was that the sensory deprivation in the visual system was associated with active sensory hallucinations in that system. Presumably, he would eventually accommodate to this and the symptoms would be expected to subside.

◆ **Diagnosis: Axis I—Alcohol Dependence, 303.90; Major Depressive Disorder, Recurrent, Severe Without Psychotic Features, 296.33; Delirium, 293.0**

Psychosomatic medicine psychiatrists treating the acute onset of bilateral blindness should be alert to this phenomenon of sensory deprivation–associated visual hallucinations. Whether this is understood as part of an experience of delirium or as a more focal psychotic symptom (as in our case) is dependent on the specifics of the case. For persistent symptoms, empirical use of antipsychotics should be considered. Helping patients deal with the trauma of their loss of vision may be complicated by the fact that they have experienced a life-changing self-inflicted disability.

Posttraumatic Stress Disorder, Electroconvulsive Therapy, and Amnesia

The patient was a 65-year-old male from Afghanistan who spoke only Farsi. As a young man in Afghanistan, he was a school teacher. During a period of political instability in his native country, he was captured by an opposing political group and brutally tortured, including having had his nails forcibly removed. Thereafter, he had had insomnia, flashbacks, nightmares, depression, paranoid ideation, anxiety and hyperarousability. He later moved to India and then eventually to the United States. Unable to work because of his lingering psychological symptoms, he spent much of his time at his family's home, where a large and involved extended family cared for and supported him. He had never learned to speak English; his adult children acted as language interpreters in his clinical care. He had been treated with various psychotropic medications with nominal improvement and was later referred for electroconvulsive therapy (ECT).

He was treated with a course of ECT, which he received as an outpatient. At the time of the ECT, he was also treated with lamotrigine 100 mg daily and olanzapine 2.5 mg twice a day. According to family observers, he began to improve after the 10th to 12th treatment session with ECT and appeared less anxious and depressed. His olanzapine was increased to 10 mg twice daily around the time of the 12th ECT session. ECT was continued; however, after his 14th session, he developed acute mental status changes. Previously capable of good cognitive function despite his profound psychological symptoms, he suddenly was confused and disoriented. He was unable to identify the time and place and told family members that he was suddenly "back in India." He became motorically agitated, and family members were not able to handle him at home. His large and caring extended family, quite aware of his history of torture and resultant lingering psychological suffering, had never encountered this behavior before. Alarmed, his family members called an ambulance service and he was brought to the emergency department.

When seen in the emergency department by the psychosomatic medicine team, he was noted to be alert, with reasonable eye contact. He spoke only through family members, two of whom commented on how he suddenly "wasn't making sense." He was anxious and dysphoric and made reference to unspecified malevolent others threatening him. Abruptly during the interview, he twice got up and walked out of the emergency department only to be later gingerly guided back by the family members to complete the interview. He was neither suicidal nor homicidal but verbalized strong themes of paranoia and confusion. His Mini-Mental State Examination (MMSE; Folstein et al. 1975) score was 11, including extremely poor orientation for time and place and severely impaired memory and concentration.

Computed tomography scans of the patient's head were unremarkable. His creatinine phosphokinase (CPK) level was normal, as were his other screening laboratories. He was admitted to the general medicine service for observation, olanzapine and lamotrigine were held, and he was treated with as-needed antipsychotic medication only. The first night in the hospital, he became agitated in the evening, struck out at nursing staff, and tried to flee the hospital, despite the presence of family members around the clock. He received a total of 24 mg of haloperidol intravenously in the first several hours of hospitalization. By the next day, he was notably calmer and showed no further agitated behavior. He thereafter did well, with gradually improving cognitive function; notably, his orientation improved substantially. His confusion and agitation did not recur. His lamotrigine was resumed, and he was started on aripiprazole 5 mg daily with close clinical follow-up. His course of ECT was not continued.

♦ **Diagnosis: Axis I—Cognitive Disorder Not Otherwise Specified (Presumptively Due to the Acute Effects of Electroconvulsive Therapy), 294.9; Posttraumatic Stress Disorder, 309.81**

This man's case was tragic and long-standing, and his experience of torture, imprisonment, with lingering traumatic memories, nightmares, flashbacks, insomnia, depression, anxiety, and hyperarousability makes chronic posttraumatic stress disorder (PTSD) the parsimonious diagnosis to explain his chronic psychological symptoms. Compounding this man's experience was the forced emigration from his country of origin and a series of moves that eventually landed him in the United States. However, his lack of English skills made him unemployable, and his continued suffering from PTSD made him capable of only minimal social function. Fortunately, he had a supportive family who provided for his needs and took care of him.

When his psychological symptoms were persistent despite medication treatment, he was treated with a course of ECT, to which he initially responded well. However, after the 14th treatment he developed acute mental status changes. These mental status changes were primarily characterized by cognitive symptoms, including disturbing disorientation and amnesia. This was associated with agitated and threatening behavior. His family, well informed of his PTSD symptoms, clearly recognized this presentation as something quite different and sought emergency care.

Amnesia after ECT is a well-recognized phenomenon. It is generally transient but nonetheless can present with acute cognitive impairment that can be quite frightening to the patient and family members. In this man's case, the concurrent dosage increase in olanzapine from 5 mg to 20 mg daily may have contributed to his decompensation, because olanzapine may have anticholinergic effects, particularly at higher doses. The combination of increased anticholinergic effect and the amnestic effects of the 14 sessions of ECT may have conspired to acutely compromise this man's cognitive function. Aripiprazole is largely devoid of anticholinergic effects, and it was chosen as an alternative medication with this concern in mind. Should this man receive further ECT, attention to the possibility of future episodes of amnesia would be necessary and critical.

Neurosarcoidosis and Psychotic Symptoms

The patient was a 50-year-old African American female with a history of stimulant abuse and psychotic disorder. She presented with acute-onset psychosis consisting of incoherent thought processes, auditory hallucinations, and delusions. She was initially admitted to a psychiatric facility. She was treated with risperidone 2 mg twice daily with minimal progress over several days; however, she developed postural instability and fell. She was emergently sent to a university medical center for evaluation.

A computed tomography scan of the head revealed a large round mass (1.5 cm in diameter) in the right frontal lobe and small lesions in the area of the nucleus accumbens. Chest x-ray revealed bilateral hilar adenopathy and pulmonary infiltrates. Brain biopsy confirmed neurosarcoidosis. On initial psychosomatic medicine consultation she had a variable level of consciousness, affective blunting, delusions, auditory hallucinations, thought disorganization, disorientation, and stereotypies. She was treated with a combination of corticosteroids (initially intravenous dexamethasone, later oral prednisone) and risperidone (titrated to 6 mg/day).

One week after she started dexamethasone, her psychiatric examination was substantially improved. She now had full level of consciousness but had continued blunted affect and continued auditory hallucinations. Her orientation was improved, but her MMSE score was 14. Over the next 10 days, she gradually resolved her psychotic symptoms; by hospital day 16, she had no further hallucinations or delusions and scored 27 on the MMSE. She had mild affective blunting and mild abulia. Repeated magnetic resonance imaging scans showed an interval decrease in the number and degree of the cortical lesions. She was discharged in stable condition.

◆ **Diagnosis: Axis I—Delirium, 293.0; Psychotic Disorder Not Otherwise Specified, 298.9; Amphetamine Abuse, 305.70**

This case illustrates how acute-onset psychosis can be due to a structural lesion, even in a patient with a history of substance abuse or other psychiatric illness. The patient responded well to combined therapy with risperidone and corticosteroids. Empirical treatment of psychosis with antipsychotics while other medications are used to treat the likely causative underlying central nervous system (CNS) lesion may be indicated to optimize clinical outcomes.

CNS illnesses such as neurosarcoidosis should be considered in acute presentations of psychotic illness; the routine use of neuroimaging in initial presentation of psychotic illness is to be encouraged. This case was complicated by the co-occurrence of psychosis and substance abuse; it may have been possible to attribute the psychotic presentation to the effects of substances. However, when the patient failed to robustly respond to initial treatment with risperidone and inpatient observation (where she did not have access to drugs), other explanations for psychosis became necessary. This need was further potentiated when she developed postural instability.

The "parallel" treatment with antipsychotics and immune-modulating corticosteroids was associated with reversal of her cognitive impairment and amelioration of her psychosis. Of course, the differential impact of these medications on her recovery is indeterminate. In such a case, the role and duration of maintenance antipsychotics remains unclear; further clinical follow-up with eventual cautious tapering of antipsychotic medication after a substantial period of clinical improvement may be warranted. Obviously, vigilance for recurrence or progression of the neurosarcoidosis itself must be maintained as well. In summary, this ambiguous case illustrates a "chicken-egg" dilemma among stimulant use, functional psychiatric illness, and structural CNS lesions as possible causative agents in the acute presentation of psychosis.

Hyperammonemia and Delirium With Valproate

We have seen cases of delirium with elevated serum ammonia due to valproate use. The elevation in serum ammonia, especially when profound and/or acute, can be associated with delirium; indeed, this delirium episode may well be the main focus of initial clinical attention.

Case 1

The first patient was a 60-year-old woman with a complex history of bipolar, anxiety, and seizure disorders who had been receiving divalproex sodium 250 mg three times a day for several months; her mood symptoms were under good control and she had had no recent seizure activity. Her other medications included diazepam 5 mg four times a day and trazodone 100 mg at bedtime. Her history was also notable for hypothyroidism (on thyroxine replacement), hypertension, fibromyalgia, chronic pain, traumatic brain injury after a motor vehicle accident, and cerebral aneurysm; the seizure disorder had developed following neurosurgical repair of the aneurysm.

Despite the complex history, she had been stable for several months with no significant medication changes. However, according to her family, she had then developed subacute mental status changes over a period of several days prior to admission. She presented to the emergency department with confusion, incoherent speech, variable level of consciousness, ataxia with falling, and amnesia. On examination, she had a variable level of consciousness and cognitive impairment. She was unable to recall recent events in her life. She was neither hypomanic/manic nor depressed, and she was not psychotic.

Initial screening laboratory results were unremarkable, including a therapeutic serum valproate level (75 mg/L). Liver-associated enzymes showed only mildly increased aspartate aminotransferase of 50 U/L; computed tomography scanning revealed only cortical volume loss that was "mildly increased for age" and evidence of past craniotomy with right frontal lobe encephalomalacia. Cerebrospinal fluid analysis was normal. Serum acetaminophen and alcohol levels were negative. Her CPK level was 1,541 U/L, and her myoglobin level was 550 ng/mL. She was admitted to the intensive care unit, and diazepam and trazodone were held. An electroencephalogram confirmed likely epileptiform activity.

Seeking to explain her presentation, the team ordered a serum ammonia level be taken; this was found to be 99 μmol/L. Her divalproex sodium was then discontinued, and levetiracetam was started in its place for seizure management. She did not receive lactulose or carnitine during her hospitalization. Within 3 days, her delirium and hyperammonemia had improved. She had returned to her baseline mental status by hospital day 6, with an MMSE score of 27; at this point her ammonia level had decreased to 48 μmol/L and her CPK level had decreased to 457 U/L. She was discharged in stable condition, instructed not to take divalproex sodium, and continued on levetiracetam for her seizure disorder.

◆ **Diagnosis: Axis I—Delirium, 293.0; Mood Disorder Not Otherwise Specified, 296.90; Anxiety Disorder Not Otherwise Specified, 300.00**

Case 2

The second case was more dramatic and acute. The patient was a 30-year-old woman with a complex psychiatric history including PTSD, bulimia nervosa, bipolar disorder, and borderline personality disorder. She had had many psychiatric hospitalizations and a complex psychopharmacological regimen. She had recently been hospitalized at a psychiatric inpatient facility, where she was stabilized on clonazepam 0.5 mg three times a day, venlafaxine extended release 225 mg daily, mirtazapine 15 mg at bedtime, bupropion sustained release 300 mg daily, and divalproex sodium 1,500 mg at bedtime; the divalproex sodium had been started near the end of her psychiatric hospitalization.

Within 2 days of discharge from the psychiatric hospital, she developed severe acute mental status changes. She became lethargic and ataxic. She was grossly confused and stopped taking food and drink. When evaluated in the field by emergency medical technicians, she was minimally responsive.

She was brought to a university medical center for evaluation. When seen in the emergency department, she had a serum ammonia level of 283 μmol/L, normal liver-associated enzyme levels and platelet counts, and a serum valproate level of 120 mg/L. Toxicology was otherwise positive only for clonazepam. Divalproex sodium and all other psychotropic medications were held; carnitine 3,000 mg intravenously and then 990 mg three times a day and lactulose 30 cc every 6 hours were started.

Within 48 hours, her hyperammonemia had resolved and her delirium had cleared. On psychosomatic medicine interview after her initial delirium had improved, she had a full level of consciousness, normal speech, organized thought processes, and an MMSE score of 25. She thereafter remained in stable condition. Her ammonia gradually decreased to 30 μmol/L by hospital day 4, at which point she was discharged. She was restarted on her other psychotropic medications (except for divalproex sodium) and discharged to outpatient care. She was to continue lactulose and carnitine for 3 days after discharge.

◆ **Diagnosis: Axis I—Delirium, 293.0; Posttraumatic Stress Disorder, 309.81; Bulimia Nervosa, 307.51; Bipolar Disorder Not Otherwise Specified, 296.80; Axis II— Borderline Personality Disorder, 301.83**

Both of these cases represent acute delirium associated with hyperammonemia (Gerster et al. 2006). Hyperammonemia is a known metabolic side effect of divalproex sodium and, unless associated with delirium, is likely benign in most cases. However, when one confronts a case of acute delirium in a patient with previous treatment with divalproex sodium, this relationship must be considered. Obviously, the patient may be receiving divalproex sodium for a purely "neurological" indication rather than a "psychiatric" one. Quite routinely, one sees physicians assiduously draw serum valproate levels, liver-associated enzymes, and platelets when evaluating patients receiving divalproex sodium; these were unremarkable in both of these cases. Evaluation of serum ammonia may require specific forethought, because many routine laboratory panels do not include ammonia levels with liver-associated enzyme panels.

As in Case 2, empirical use of carnitine is considered for extreme elevation in serum ammonia; as needed, this can be combined with lactulose. As psychiatrists continue to routinely use divalproex sodium for numerous psychiatric illnesses, the possibility of iatrogenic hyperammonemia should be kept in mind, especially when previously well-compensated divalproex sodium–treated patients present with delirium. When encountering this presentation, clinicians should consider routine screening of ammonia levels and collaborate in appropriately assertive management of this toxic state.

Adjunctive Valproic Acid for Delirium and/or Agitation

Conventional management of delirium typically involves the use of antipsychotic agents, with benzodiazepines used in a supplementary role or as primary therapy for delirium associated with sedative, hypnotic, or alcohol withdrawal. Mastery of delirium management, despite the relative paucity of randomized, controlled studies, remains a major area of clinical skill in psychosomatic medicine. However, there are particular cases in which conventional delirium management with antipsychotics and benzodiazepines is associated either with limited clinical success or with medication side effects that make the clinician search for other clinical interventions. Although anecdotal, there may be a place for the supplemental use of valproate, which is already in common use for bipolar disorders and other agitated states. Our group has reported on six cases of supplemental use of valproate for delirium and/or agitation (Bourgeois et al. 2005).

Case 1

The first case was that of a 45-year-old white male with a history of alcohol dependence who presented with an acute surgical abdomen with peritonitis and underwent an emergency laparotomy. He was found to have a gastric ulcer, and he received an antrectomy and gastrojejunostomy. Postoperatively, he developed respiratory distress (requiring intubation and ventilation, and bronchoscopy to remove mucous plugs) and ventricular fibrillation (requiring defibrillation). He developed delirium in the context of these postoperative complications. Delirium symptoms included agitation, sleep-wake cycle disturbances, variable level of consciousness, and psychosis. His agitation was largely unresponsive to several psychopharmacological agents, including benzodiazepines and haloperidol; haloperidol was also associated with prolongation of his QT_c interval and was discontinued. The prolonged QT_c interval was particularly worrisome because of his having had an episode of ventricular fibrillation. A further challenge was his development of an enterocutaneous fistula, which required a prolonged period of nothing-by-mouth status.

Psychosomatic medicine consultation was then obtained. Examination findings included variable level of consciousness, agitated behavior, poor orientation, persecutory delusions, and auditory and visual hallucinations. He was started on intravenous valproate sodium 500 mg twice daily and lorazepam 1 mg four times a day. Within 3 days he was less agitated and more cognitively organized, with intact orientation to time, place, and person as well as improved short-term memory and concentration. His lorazepam was then tapered with further mental status improvement, and he had an MMSE score of 29 within 10 days of starting the valproate sodium.

◆ **Diagnosis: Axis I—Alcohol Dependence, 303.90;
Delirium, 293.0**

Case 2

The patient was a 47-year-old white male with a history of esophageal carcinoma, status postesophagectomy with gastric pull-up, chemotherapy, pneumonitis, persistent fevers, pulmonary edema, hepatitis C, and peptic ulcer disease. He had an acute upper gastrointestinal bleed requiring arterial embolization and transfusion.

He also had treatment for bacteremia and fungemia and required intubation and ventilatory support.

Psychosomatic medicine consultation was requested to manage agitation and altered level of consciousness. Because of his delirium, he could not be weaned from the ventilator. At the time of consultation, he was receiving lorazepam 1 mg intravenously every hour and hydromorphone 6 mg every hour. He was then started on haloperidol 2.5 mg intravenously every 8 hours and diazepam 5 mg intravenously every 6 hours; lorazepam was discontinued. His agitation then decreased somewhat, and he was able to respond to questions by "mouthing" his answers. In view of his continued delirium, his haloperidol was increased to 5 mg intravenously every 6 hours. Despite this dosage increase, he continued to have breakthrough agitation. Liquid valproate 250 mg every 6 hours by nasogastric tube was then added and diazepam was discontinued. After he presented with a prolonged QT_c interval, haloperidol was discontinued. Four days after initiation of valproate, his agitation was well controlled, his level of consciousness fluctuations improved, and his ability to communicate was increased.

◆ **Diagnosis: Axis I—Delirium, 293.0**

Case 3

The patient was a 50-year-old white male with obstructive sleep apnea, chronic obstructive pulmonary disorder, morbid obesity, hypoventilation syndrome, congestive heart failure, diabetes mellitus, venous thrombosis, depression, and PTSD. He was admitted after further compromise of his respiratory status; he developed pneumonia and was treated with antibiotics. He also experienced a gastrointestinal bleed that required transfusions. He was treated with diazepam 20 mg intravenously every 4 hours, paroxetine 40 mg by nasogastric tube daily, and fluphenazine 5 mg by nasogastric tube every 6 hours. Despite this regimen, he had continued breakthrough agitation and received frequent as-needed doses of midazolam and lorazepam. A psychosomatic medicine consultation was obtained for management of continued agitation.

On examination, he had a variable level of consciousness, hallucinations, and confusion. He was oriented in three spheres. He was begun on oral liquid valproate 575 mg three times a day, risperidone 2 mg every 6 hours, lorazepam 2 mg every 6 hours, and sertraline 50 mg daily, all delivered via nasogastric tube; diazepam, paroxetine, and fluphenazine were stopped. Over the next few days, his agitation and sleep pattern substantially improved; lorazepam was then held.

His QT$_c$ interval was noted to have increased to 470 msec; risperidone was then held as well. His valproate dosage was increased to 650 mg by nasogastric tube three times a day and his sertraline was eventually increased to 150 mg daily. His agitation remained under control and he was then able to tolerate ventilatory weaning trials without agitation.

◆ **Diagnosis: Axis I—Posttraumatic Stress Disorder, 309.81; Major Depressive Disorder, Recurrent, Severe Without Psychotic Features, 296.33; Delirium, 293.0**

Case 4

The patient was a 40-year-old white male with a history of bipolar disorder, for which he had received lithium carbonate 1,800 mg daily. He was admitted after a complicated case of pneumonia that led to his requiring intubation and ventilation for respiratory distress. Initially, his lithium carbonate was continued during his hospitalization. However, his mental status deteriorated to include waxing and waning level of consciousness, intermittent agitation, and periods of excessive somnolence. On examination, he was sedated, briefly arousable, and only able to follow simple directions. Lithium was discontinued and liquid valproate 750 mg by nasogastric tube three times a day was started; because of his continued agitation, the evening dosage was later increased to 1,000 mg. On this dosage of valproate, his agitation was notably improved, but he still had occasional episodes of breakthrough agitation. Risperidone 2 mg every 6 hours and lorazepam 1 mg every 6 hours were added, both via nasogastric tube. Subsequently, his agitation did not return, his cognitive status cleared, and his level of consciousness fluctuations resolved.

◆ **Diagnosis: Axis I—Bipolar Disorder Not Otherwise Specified, 296.80; Delirium, 293.0**

Case 5

The patient was a 41-year-old white male with a history of polysubstance dependence who experienced agitation and disorganized behavior after a motor vehicle accident with multiple skeletal traumas. He then developed bacteremia and respiratory distress. As-needed doses of midazolam and fentanyl did not control his episodes of agitation. On psychosomatic medicine consultation, he was disoriented and tangential and could not provide appropriate answers. He was agitated and trying to leave his bed, despite being in traction.

Affect was anxious and labile; speech was loud, rapid, and pressured. His level of consciousness was variable, and his MMSE score was 2.

He was treated initially with haloperidol intravenously in three escalating doses of 10 mg, 20 mg, and 30 mg but did not improve. He was then treated with haloperidol 10 mg intravenously four times a day, lorazepam 3 mg intravenously every hour, and liquid valproate 250 mg by nasogastric tube twice daily. Lorazepam was then discontinued and replaced by diazepam 15 mg orally three times a day. Within 3 days of the combination therapy, his agitation was substantially improved; within 8 days, it resolved completely, his mood was improved, and his MMSE score rose to 26. Diazepam and haloperidol were tapered and valproate was continued; he remained in stable and improved condition.

◆ **Diagnosis: Axis I—Polysubstance Dependence, 304.80; Delirium, 293.0**

Case 6

The patient was a 63-year-old white male with a long history of paranoid schizophrenia. He was admitted for an esophageal rupture, which caused him to be put on persistent nothing-by-mouth status. He experienced a variable level of consciousness, agitation, suspiciousness, aggressive behavior, and refusal of needed clinical interventions. On psychosomatic medicine consultation, he was paranoid and unwilling to answer questions and cooperate with the interview. He was treated with haloperidol 5 mg intravenously at bedtime; over 2 weeks, the dosage was increased to 5 mg intravenously every morning and 10 mg intravenously at bedtime. Despite this dosage of haloperidol, he continued to be paranoid, aggressive, and hostile. Because of his mental status, he lacked the capacity to consent to a surgical procedure. He also had no surrogate to provide operative consent on his behalf. As a result, he was to be on nothing-by-mouth status indefinitely. Because of his continued agitation, he had valproate sodium 250 mg intravenously twice daily added to his regimen; this dosage was increased to 500 mg intravenously every 6 hours. Within several days of starting valproate, he was much less agitated and more cooperative with medical care and procedures. His mood lability also improved markedly.

◆ **Diagnosis: Axis I—Schizophrenia, Paranoid Type, 295.30; Delirium, 293.0**

These cases illustrate patients with varying degrees of agitation associated with delirium that were only incompletely responsive to conventional psychopharmacology for delirium. In each case, adjunctive use of oral or intravenous valproate was associated with less agitation and improvement in delirium. In patients whose illness is refractory to conventional management or in whom conventional agents are poorly tolerated, the creative and judicious use (under the appropriate monitoring of laboratory parameters) of valproate might eventually represent a "third pathway" in the treatment of delirium, corresponding to the "first and second pathways" of antipsychotics and benzodiazepines, respectively.

Neuroleptic Malignant Syndrome Vigilance

NMS, although an uncommon problem in most psychiatric practices, is an illness of major importance in psychosomatic medicine (Gurrera 1999). The classic presentation of hyperthermia, "lead-pipe" muscle rigidity, altered mental status, and extremely high CPK level in a patient treated with antipsychotic agents is unmistakable (Caroff and Mann 1993; Levenson 1985). However, more subtle presentations also happen and, paradoxically, could lead to poor clinical outcomes because of their less dramatic appearance and resultant diagnostic and interventional nihilism on the part of treating physicians. We have seen several cases that illustrate this point. Notably, all of these cases were associated with atypical antipsychotic medications, which may be categorically associated with a milder form of NMS, perhaps related to the more modest degrees of dopamine D_2 blockade associated with these agents compared with typical antipsychotic agents (Hasan and Buckley 1998).

Case 1

The first patient was a 40-year-old white female with a long and complex psychiatric history. She was the survivor of childhood abuse and neglect and first experienced psychotic symptoms in her early 20s. She had been psychiatrically hospitalized many times, including state hospital commitment, had had a legal conservator appointed, and had been treated with a complex series of psychotropic medications. Notably, she had had NMS on three prior occasions; each of

these prior NMS episodes had been associated with typical antipsychotic agents.

She had recently been psychiatrically hospitalized for yet another
time; she had then been stabilized and discharged on a regimen that
included quetiapine 50 mg every morning and 150 mg at bedtime;
clozapine 400 mg, divalproex sodium 750 mg, and lamotrigine
200 mg, all at bedtime; and clonazepam 2 mg twice a day. The other
medications had been stable for months in terms of dosage and frequency; only the quetiapine was newly added during this last psychiatric hospitalization.

Shortly after having been discharged from the psychiatric hospital, she developed increased temperature and altered mental status.
She was admitted with the following findings: temperature 101.0°F,
muscle rigidity, tachycardia, agitation, decreased cognition, and a
CPK level of 1,128 U/L. Antipsychotics were held and she was
resuscitated with intravenous fluids in the intensive care unit. Her
CPK level peaked at 2,568 U/L, and bromocriptine 1.25 mg orally
twice a day was started. As her delirium cleared and she was extubated, she verbalized paranoid delusions. Her CPK level decreased
to 665 U/L by hospital day 4 and to 60 U/L 10 days later. She was
transferred in stable condition to the psychiatric facility. Clozapine,
divalproex sodium, lamotrigine, and clonazepam were restarted, but
quetiapine was not resumed; the NMS did not subsequently recur.

◆ **Diagnosis: Axis I—Psychotic Disorder Not Otherwise
Specified, 298.9; Neuroleptic Malignant Syndrome,
333.92**

This was a complex case, both historically and at clinical presentation. Because the balance of her chronic psychotropic medication
regimen had been well tolerated without the signs of NMS, it appeared that this NMS episode was precipitated by the addition of
quetiapine. Notably, the dosage of quetiapine was itself relatively
modest, and quetiapine has only rarely been associated with NMS.
In addition, the co-administration of clozapine (itself of minimal
NMS risk but perhaps representing some additive risk with other
psychotropic medications) and two anticonvulsants (divalproex sodium and lamotrigine) may have increased the risk of NMS when
quetiapine was later introduced. It has been occasionally reported
that co-administration of antipsychotic agents with anticonvulsants
may increase the risk of NMS through an as yet obscure mechanism.
Finally, this patient, although clearly rigid, delirious, and quite ill,

never manifested a dramatic elevation of CPK; her peak CPK level was 2,568 U/L. Therefore, vigilance for NMS, guided by the patient's prior episodes of NMS, the presence of two antipsychotics (each independently associated with a low risk of NMS by themselves), and the co-administration of two anticonvulsants were possible additive factors in this case.

Case 2

The second patient was a 33-year-old white male with a history of bipolar disorder. He was admitted to the medical center on urgent transfer from a psychiatric hospital for acute onset of tachycardia, labile blood pressure, hyperthermia, confusion, and withdrawn social behavior. Ten days previously, he had been switched from his habitual regimen of combined olanzapine and divalproex to combined risperidone and lithium carbonate. He had previously been clinically stable in terms of psychiatric symptoms but had had substantial weight gain on olanzapine and divalproex; hence the motivation for these medication changes. He had had no prior episodes of NMS.

On examination, he was hypertensive (189/101 mm Hg) and tachycardic (174 beats per minute), and his temperature was 102.3°F. He had altered and fluctuating level of consciousness, auditory hallucinations, muscle fasciculations, and rigidity. His blood urea nitrogen and creatinine levels were increased; CPK level was 1,428 U/L. He was diagnosed with NMS; antipsychotics were held, and lithium was discontinued. He received as-needed lorazepam for tremors and agitation. Over several days, his mental status, rigidity, and CPK and other laboratory values returned to normal. He was transferred to a psychiatric hospital on day 6 for definitive inpatient psychiatric care.

◆ **Diagnosis: Axis I—Bipolar I Disorder, Most Recent Episode Unspecified, 296.7; Neuroleptic Malignant Syndrome, 333.92**

This patient showed manifestations of NMS within several days of beginning therapy with risperidone and lithium. Notably, the patient had tolerated a similar combined regimen of olanzapine and divalproex without prior episodes of NMS. The peak CPK level was only 1,428 U/L, but his autonomic instability and physical signs made the diagnosis clear. With attentive, supportive management he improved quickly. Clinicians should be particularly attentive to the NMS risk when antipsychotic medications are changed, particularly if there is concurrently a new mood stabilizer initiated.

Case 3

A third case illustrated the NMS risk of the new antipsychotic aripiprazole. The patient was a 23-year-old white female with a recent onset of psychotic disorder with dramatic persecutory delusions and hallucinations. She had been a user of methamphetamine, but the psychiatric facility treating her could not definitively establish a causal relationship between her drug use and the onset of the psychotic illness. She was started on aripiprazole 30 mg every morning during a brief psychiatric inpatient admission. On aripiprazole, her psychosis cleared. She promptly stabilized and was discharged.

Two weeks later, she presented emergently to the emergency department with tremors, rigidity, and diaphoresis. On examination, she manifested agitation, tremors, rigidity, diaphoresis, and altered mental status. Her temperature was 100.0°F, her blood pressure was variable between 109–135/72–79 mm Hg, and she was tachycardic (up to 118 beats per minute). She had mild leukocytosis (14 K/mm^3) and a CPK of 866 U/L.

She was admitted and treated for presumptive NMS; aripiprazole was held, and she received as-needed doses of lorazepam. She was also treated with bromocriptine 2.5 mg twice daily for the rigidity. Her CPK level gradually normalized, and her mental status cleared. Her rigidity and tremor resolved by hospital day 5. She exhibited recurrence of delusional thoughts after medical stabilization and was transferred to a psychiatric facility after 9 days of hospitalization.

◆ **Diagnosis: Axis I—Amphetamine Abuse, 305.70;**
  Psychotic Disorder Not Otherwise Specified, 298.9;
  Neuroleptic Malignant Syndrome, 333.92

This case illustrates how NMS can develop early in the course of treatment with aripiprazole. Notably, the patient's peak CPK level was only 866 U/L; a level that could have been attributed to other nonspecific factors. Once identified as NMS, she resolved with supportive and symptomatic treatment. Vigilance for NMS needs to include cases with the newest antipsychotics and the early phase of treatment; conceivably, the aggressive dosing strategy of early use of the 30 mg daily dose of aripiprazole in this patient may have unwittingly contributed to the risk of the NMS episode.

Case 4

Another case of early-onset NMS occurred in a teenage patient, with remarkably rapid onset of NMS following antipsychotic and mood stabilizer combination therapy. The patient was a 17-year-old African American male with a recent onset of a manic episode with psychotic features. He had an abrupt onset of rapid and pressured speech, a decreased need for sleep, increased physical energy, disorganized thoughts, hallucinations, and delusions. He was admitted to a psychiatric facility for stabilization. After admission to the psychiatric facility, he was started on olanzapine 7.5 mg daily and divalproex sodium 750 mg daily. Within 24 hours of the beginning of this combination therapy, he had a temperature of 101.2°F, pulse of 148 beats per minute, diaphoresis, decreased level of consciousness, and a CPK level of 2,288 U/L.

He was emergently transferred to the medical center, where he displayed motor agitation, waxy flexibility, and rigidity. A repeated CPK level was 4,650 U/L. He required intubation and mechanical ventilation and was started on dantrolene and aggressive hydration. He stabilized over the next 6 days and was extubated. During this time, his CPK level normalized, and his motor signs improved. However, he continued to exhibit paranoid ideation and minimal social interactions, despite stabilization of his mood state. He was started on clozapine and was transferred to the psychiatric hospital for definitive psychiatric care.

♦ **Diagnosis: Axis I—Schizophreniform Disorder, 295.40; Neuroleptic Malignant Syndrome, 333.92**

The abrupt onset of severe NMS within hours of combination antipsychotic/mood stabilizer therapy in this case was most striking. There was nothing in the history to suggest that this unfortunate boy was at particular risk of NMS; he had no previous psychiatric history, his dosages of psychotropic medications were routine and appeared appropriate for his clinical condition, and he was in a contained inpatient psychiatric environment with regular observation. Prompt emergency evaluation and management on the intensive care unit resolved his NMS episode. Not unexpectedly, he remained psychotic when he recovered from the NMS episode. Among the various choices to treat his residual psychosis, it was believed that clozapine (manifesting minimal D_2 blockade among the atypical antipsychotic agents) offered the lowest risk of another NMS episode, albeit with the usual requirements for monitoring for agranulocytosis.

The classic presentation of NMS is unmistakable, but in the current clinical environment, with the routine use of atypical antipsychotic agents, a more subtle presentation may be encountered. Significant (but not grossly dramatic) muscle rigidity, clearly elevated CPK levels in the 1,000–3,000 U/L range, autonomic instability, and recent first exposure to antipsychotic agents may be seen. In addition, the physician should be especially vigilant for NMS cases with concurrent use of antipsychotics and anticonvulsants. Finally, patients with clear prior episodes of NMS (or illness episodes phenomenologically similar to NMS, in retrospect) should be approached with particular caution.

Serotonin Syndrome Versus Neuroleptic Malignant Syndrome: A False Dichotomy or an Ambiguous Presentation?

The distinction between serotonin syndrome and NMS may be a challenging one, because the clinical phenomenology overlap substantially and both are often consequent to use of psychotropic medications (Boyer and Shannon 2005; Sternbach 1991). Indeed, some cases may be parsimoniously conceptualized on a "continuum" between these two admittedly somewhat amorphously defined, yet clinically potentially dangerous, conditions. The physical, neurological, and mental status examinations may offer some insight but may also be as "amorphous" as the phenomenological and conceptual constructs of these illnesses. Notably, perhaps reflecting its relatively recent description in the literature, serotonin syndrome is not even listed in the DSM-IV-TR diagnoses. Adding to psychiatrists' concerns is that these conditions are usually considered iatrogenic because they are often the consequence of the use of psychotropic medications. The psychiatrist may feel a particular obligation to identify and properly manage these illnesses, because our specialty may well be often responsible for the psychopharmacological treatment that occasionally results in these illnesses.

The examination findings of these two conditions have much in common. Patients are typically delirious, but the type of delirium (hypoactive, hyperactive, or mixed), although routinely useful to classify and describe, does not reliably distinguish between these conditions. The NMS patient may, at presentation, have more profound delirium and a lower level of consciousness, whereas serotonin syndrome patients tend to be more hyperaroused (Boyer and Shannon 2005). However, this distinction is at best a qualitative one and must be corroborated by other observations and clinical findings. Similarly, although both illnesses present with increased muscular tone, NMS patients are more likely to be grossly "lead-pipe" rigid than serotonin syndrome patients. One physical finding that may distinguish between serotonin syndrome and NMS are deep tendon reflexes, which should be routinely examined in acutely delirious and rigid patients with access to psychotropic medications. NMS patients typically have either normal or decreased deep tendon reflexes (proportional to the degree of muscle rigidity), whereas serotonin syndrome patients will classically have hyperreflexia or even clonus (Boyer and Shannon 2005).

The history may provide for a distinction between serotonin syndrome and NMS with some validity, although patients with complex psychopharmacology regimens may be at risk for both disorders. Serotonin syndrome patients will have had access to serotonergic medications (e.g., psychotropic medications such as selective serotonin reuptake inhibitors, serotonin norepinephrine reuptake inhibitors, trazodone, buspirone, and monoamine oxidase inhibitors) as well as other medications generally used for nonpsychiatric indications such as selegiline and tramadol (Boyer and Shannon 2005). Often there has been a recent dosage increase or addition of another serotonergic medication to the patient's regimen. Not infrequently, depressed or personality-disordered patients make suicide attempts with large doses of serotonergic psychotropic agents; this can, of course, also result in serotonin syndrome. Another possible scenario precipitating an episode of serotonin syndrome is the previously stable patient receiving serotonergic psychotropic medications who then experiences decreased hepatic metabolism of the serotonergic medications, for example, the depressed alcohol-dependent patient with progressive hepatic failure.

In distinction to the aforementioned psychotropic agents, atypical antipsychotic agents typically do not cause serotonin syndrome (in fact, they are sometimes recommended as an intervention for serotonin syndrome) (Boyer and Shannon 2005). This is probably because their serotonin effects are postsynaptic at the serotonin 5-HT_2 receptor. Atypical antipsychotics are increasingly recognized, of course, as causative of NMS (although probably at a risk lower than that of typical antipsychotic agents) because of their property of D_2 receptor blockade.

A 35-year-old male with a history of depression with psychotic features and chronic pain had been treated as an outpatient with citalopram, buspirone, and olanzapine; he recently had had his citalopram increased for recurrence of depressive symptoms. Shortly thereafter, he developed sweating, increased temperature, clouding of consciousness, mild rigidity, and constitutional symptoms of fatigue and myalgia. Upon examination, he was delirious, with mild rigidity and mildly increased CPK level. His deep tendon reflexes were increased without clonus.

Was this condition serotonin syndrome or mild NMS? Given the lack of a definitive laboratory test to distinguish between the two conditions, this distinction was difficult. He had had exposure to both "high-risk" groups of medications: a serotonergic antidepressant and serotonergic anxiolytic that additively increased the risk for serotonin syndrome and an atypical antipsychotic that increased the risk for NMS. He was clearly rigid but not grossly so; severe "lead-pipe" rigidity is consistent with severe, classic NMS. Similarly, his CPK level was elevated, but not to alarmingly high levels. He was hyperreflexic (suggesting serotonin syndrome) but did not have spontaneous clonus (which would be more specific for serotonin syndrome).

Psychosomatic medicine management simultaneously pursued both possibilities; temporarily treating him as though he had both serotonin syndrome and NMS. Citalopram, buspirone, and olanzapine were all held when he was admitted. He was admitted to the intensive care unit and intravenously hydrated. Breakthrough episodes of agitation were treated with cautious dosing of lorazepam; antipsychotic agents were avoided. Mental status examination and physical examination for rigidity and reflexes were accomplished daily, and his CPK level and renal panel were examined daily. Over a period of several days, his delirium, rigidity, and CPK level all cleared. He never developed clonus, and his hyperreflexia had resolved.

◆ **Diagnosis: Axis I—Delirium, 293.0; Rule Out Neuroleptic Malignant Syndrome, 333.92; Rule Out Serotonin Syndrome (No DSM-IV-TR Code)**

In ambiguous cases of serotonin syndrome versus neuroleptic malignant syndrome, the dichotomous choice between these conditions may indeed be a false one. This patient presented with evidence of both conditions, which have overlapping physical findings with each other. The diagnostic imprecision may initially lead to a clinical management dilemma. Approaching such cases in a manner that allows the clinician to entertain one or both diagnoses may be the best approach. Supportive care, withdrawal of putatively causative agents, frequent mental status examination, relevant neurological examination, and appropriate laboratory assessments as though both conditions were present may be the safest course of action.

An Ambiguous Toxicology Case

A middle-aged white man was found by city police to be staggering near railroad tracks and was taken to an acute psychiatric crisis unit for evaluation of his odd behavior. At the psychiatric crisis unit, the patient was noted to be motorically agitated, hypertensive, and tachycardic. He was transferred to the emergency department of a university medical center for assessment. In the emergency department, the patient was given a total of 20 mg intramuscular haloperidol, 10 mg intramuscular ziprasidone, and 20 mg intravenous lorazepam for control of acute agitation. He also received several doses of physostigmine for presumed anticholinergic toxicity before being orally intubated for airway protection. He was admitted to the intensive care unit, and the psychosomatic medicine service was consulted for management of his agitation and altered mental status. On initial evaluation, the patient had just been extubated but was unable to give any useful information. The patient's father provided the critical collateral history that the patient had a history of substance abuse, most notably alcohol, and a history of schizophrenia, for which he took quetiapine, escitalopram, and bupropion.

One day after admission to intensive care, the patient was confused, motorically agitated, and evidenced hyperreflexia and clonus. His pupils were dilated, his blood pressure was 170/90 mm Hg, and his heart rate was 115 beats per minute. Laboratory values included a CPK level greater than 20,000 IU/L, aspartate aminotransferase four times normal, and alanine aminotransferase twice normal. An electrocardiogram showed a prolonged QT_c interval of 470 msec. The initial differential diagnosis included serotonin syndrome, NMS, anticholinergic toxicity, and alcohol withdrawal. A gas chromatography toxicology screening was positive for quetiapine and bupropion. The patient was treated with lorazepam for presumed alcohol withdrawal. Antipsychotics were held for suspicion of NMS.

After 2 days in intensive care, the patient's mental status cleared, and he now admitted to an overdose of quetiapine (40 of the 300-mg tablets) in response to a fight with his girlfriend and removal of custody of his children. He also admitted to recent drinking of 6–12 beers per day for several months leading up to his presentation. He expressed regret for his actions but admitted to ongoing severe depression and hopelessness. His CPK level fell to less than 5,000 U/L over several days, and he tolerated a benzodiazepine taper without a recurrence of symptoms, suggesting withdrawal. Upon medical stabilization, he was sent back to the inpatient psychiatric facility for treatment.

◆ **Diagnosis: Axis I—Schizophrenia, Undifferentiated Type, 295.90; Depressive Disorder Not Otherwise Specified, 311; Alcohol Dependence, 303.90; Delirium, 293.0; Rule Out Neuroleptic Malignant Syndrome, 333.92**

This case is curious in the variety of findings associated with an overdose of the atypical antipsychotic quetiapine and the overlap of these findings with other states of delirium, including anticholinergic toxicity, NMS, serotonin syndrome, and alcohol withdrawal. Our patient did indeed have symptoms of serotonin syndrome (hypertension, tachycardia, hyperreflexia, myoclonus), NMS (autonomic instability, muscular rigidity, altered mental status, elevated CPK level), and anticholinergic toxicity (altered mental status, tachycardia). It remained unclear whether quetiapine toxicity alone could have caused all of the observed abnormalities in vital signs, laboratory values, and physical examination.

A review of 14 cases of quetiapine overdose found 3 patients with prolonged QT_c interval, 9 with tachycardia, 8 with somnolence, 4 with hypotension, and 2 with mild to moderate increases in CPK level (Hunfeld et al. 2006). A case series reviewing 18 cases of confirmed quetiapine overdose found seizures in 2 patients, prolonged QT_c interval and tachycardia in 8 of 10 patients whose electrocardiograms were included, delirium in 3 patients, and hypotension in 1 patient (Balit et al. 2003). CPK levels were not discussed in this case series. In both studies, many patients ingested other drugs in addition to quetiapine.

Although many of our patient's symptoms may have been due to quetiapine overdose, the degree of CPK elevation and muscular rigidity observed was unusual compared with other reports of quetiapine toxicity (Balit et al. 2003; Hunfeld et al. 2006). Elevated CPK level has been reported with quetiapine use *without* other signs of NMS (Klein et al. 2006). Although NMS has been reported with quetiapine (Bourgeois et al. 2002), it is more commonly associated with high-potency antipsychotics such as haloperidol. The additional antipsychotics administered in the emergency department may have played a part in the "NMS-like" presentation seen in the intensive care unit.

Another possible contributor to many of these symptoms (autonomic instability, agitation, altered mental status) could have been alcohol withdrawal. Fortunately, the treatment for many of these syndromes is the same (supportive care, benzodiazepines), and other than the initial use of physostigmine for anticholinergic toxicity, and possibly dantrolene and bromocriptine for NMS, no specific antidote to any of the possible overdoses is the current standard of care.

References

American Psychiatric Association: Diagnostic and Statistical Manual of Mental Disorders, 4th Edition, Text Revision. Washington, DC, American Psychiatric Association, 2000

Balit CB, Isbister GK, Kackett LP, et al: Quetiapine poisoning: a case series. Ann Emerg Med 42:751–758, 2003

Bourgeois JA, Babine S, Meyerovich M, et al: A case of neuroleptic malignant syndrome with quetiapine (letter). J Neuropsychiatry Clin Neurosci 14:87, 2002

Bourgeois JA, Koike AK, Simmons JE, et al: Adjunctive valproic acid for delirium and/or agitation on a consultation-liaison service: a report of six cases. J Neuropsychiatry Clin Neurosci 17:232–238, 2005

Boyer EW, Shannon M: The serotonin syndrome. N Engl J Med 352:1112–1120, 2005

Caroff SN, Mann SC: Neuroleptic malignant syndrome. Med Clin North Am 77:185–202, 1993

Folstein MF, Folstein SE, McHugh PR: "Mini-Mental State": a practical method for grading the cognitive state of patients for the clinician. J Psychiatr Res 12:189–198, 1975

Gerster T, Buesing D, Longin E, et al: Valproic acid induced encephalopathy: 19 new cases in Germany from 1994 to 2003—a side effect associated to VPA-therapy not only in young children. Seizure 15:443–448, 2006

Gurrera RJ: Sympathoadrenal hyperactivity and the etiology of neuroleptic malignant syndrome. Am J Psychiatry 156:169–180, 1999

Hasan S, Buckley P: Novel antipsychotics and the neuroleptic malignant syndrome: a review and critique. Am J Psychiatry 155:1113–1116, 1998

Hunfeld NGM, Westerman EM, Boswijk DJ, et al: Quetiapine in overdose: a clinical and pharmacokinetic analysis of 14 cases. Ther Drug Monit 28:185–189, 2006

Klein JP, Fiedler U, Appel H, et al: Massive creatine kinase elevations with quetiapine: report of two cases. Pharmacopsychiatry 39:39–40, 2006

Levenson JL: Neuroleptic malignant syndrome. Am J Psychiatry 142:1137–1145, 1985

Lonergan E, Britton AM, Luxemberg J, et al: Antipsychotics for delirium. Cochrane Database Sys Rev CD005594, 2007

Slatkin N, Rhiner M: Treatment of opiate-induced delirium with acetylcholinesterase inhibitors: a case report. J Pain Symptom Manage 27:268–273, 2004

Slatkin NE, Rhiner M, Bolton TM: Donepezil in the treatment of opioid-induced sedation: a report of six cases. J Pain Symptom Manage 21:425–438, 2001

Sternbach H: The serotonin syndrome. Am J Psychiatry 148:705–713, 1991

3

HEART DISEASE

Psychosomatic medicine psychiatrists have an inherent interest in cardiovascular disease. Acute presentation of symptomatic chest pain, thought by the patient to represent acute coronary syndrome, is often ultimately diagnosed as panic disorder. Anxiety of a more general and tonic nature is experienced with physical sensations of chronic palpitations and tachycardia. Patients with coronary artery disease have a high incidence of depression; depression in coronary artery disease has been shown to independently affect survival in these patients. Heart disease is a common illness leading to hospitalization, and these patients will often have emotional difficulties confronting the threat to physical health and survival that these illnesses often represent. Thus, comfort and familiarity with the psychiatric aspects of cardiovascular disease are regularly required in psychosomatic medicine practice.

Delirium and Vascular Dementia Diagnosed Post–Coronary Artery Bypass Graft

The post–coronary artery bypass graft (CABG) patient presenting with acute delirium is a familiar intensive care unit case in psychosomatic medicine that often graphically illustrates the complex and temporal connections between delirium and dementia; in addition, because of the common occurrence of depression in coronary artery disease, these patients often have comorbid depression (Burns et al. 2004; Litaker et al. 2001). These cases may be illustrated by the application of a "triple D triangle" in which the three points of the triangle represent dementia, delirium, and depression. Often, when one encounters such a patient acutely, the delirium presentation is the most urgent one, but the dementia and depression aspects may need to be integrated into the case formulation in a comprehensive and emerging way.

> The patient was a 65-year-old male with multiple vascular risk factors (diabetes mellitus, hypertension, hyperlipidemia, and smoking) who had presented to the medical center in unstable angina. Emergent cardiac catheterization revealed critical coronary artery disease, and the patient was taken promptly to CABG surgery. There were no surgical complications, but shortly after transfer to the intensive care unit postoperatively he experienced motor agitation (nighttime worse than daytime), confusion, disorientation (mistaking the intensive-care room for his own home and mistaking hospital personnel for his own family), and circadian rhythm disturbance.
>
> When seen in consultation the next morning, he had a variable level of consciousness, was grossly confused and disoriented, and was seeing "animals and people" in the room. He denied suicidal ideation and homicidal ideation and had a Mini-Mental State Examination (MMSE; Folstein et al. 1975) score of 12. Magnetic resonance imaging of the brain showed diffuse cortical atrophy and small-vessel white matter disease. Collateral history from family members revealed a gradual onset of mild problems with memory and word finding, without grossly impaired social function. He had also appeared to family members to have been "down" over his chronic medical illnesses and the functional limitations associated with them, with mild sleep, low energy, and appetite disturbance. He had had no formal psychiatric history and no prior psychiatric or psychotropic interventions.
>
> He was diagnosed with delirium and vascular dementia, and depression needed to be ruled out. He was treated with low-dosage antipsychotic (risperidone 0.25 mg orally twice a day) for delirium; opioids were minimized, and anticholinergic medications and benzodiazepines were held. Over the next several days, his disturbed sleep-wake cycle was corrected, his hallucinations and motor agitation resolved, and he became more accurately oriented.
>
> His repeat MMSE score was 22, with difficulties in short-term recall and concentration; mild problems with orientation to day of week, date of the month, and hospital floor number persisted. He was treated with donepezil 5 mg orally at bedtime; after several more days with no further symptoms of delirium, his risperidone was discontinued. Because his affect continued to be dysphoric, citalopram 20 mg by mouth daily was added. He was eventually dis-

charged from the hospital in stable condition; he was less dysphoric, and his final MMSE score was 26.

◆ **Diagnosis: Axis I—Delirium, 293.0; Vascular Dementia, With Depressed Mood, 290.43; Depressive Disorder Not Otherwise Specified, 311**

This case represents a case of the "three Ds." The patient had had mild depression in the context of chronic vascular disease, for which he had not previously received psychotropic medication. Sometime later (perhaps concurrently), he began to exhibit mild cognitive impairment. It is often difficult to distinguish with precision the relative contributions of untreated depression (in which mood disorders are modeled as serotonergic and/or noradrenergic phenomena) and mild vascular dementia (in which the memory and other cognitive complaints may be modeled as cholinergic phenomena) to the net functional cognitive impairment.

It is more intuitive to connect the chronic (and thus often underrecognized and undertreated) vascular dementia to the eventual development of delirium. This has been described as a problem of "diminished cognitive reserve" as a delirium risk factor. An important predictive factor for postoperative delirium is preoperative dementia, although the preoperative dementia, if clinically subtle, is often only recognized and classified retrospectively and postoperatively from the perspective of a recognized delirium case.

Management of these cases involves active examination of the three apices of the "three D triangle," with shifting attention to the various components of the case over time as clinical events unfold. At various times, the three components may vary in terms of clinical primacy. When encountering the delirious patient, management of delirium is primary, or, in other words, "delirium transcends all other psychiatric illnesses." In a case such as this one, early use of neuroimaging is helpful, not for elucidation of the delirium per se (because delirium is a clinical diagnosis, not a radiological one), but because "every delirium workup is also a dementia workup." For the evaluation of dementia, neuroimaging is a routine assessment.

The clinical management of delirium in these cases overlaps with the standard management of other delirium cases. Avoidance of anticholinergic medications, especially diphenhydramine (so as not to exacerbate the functionally evident cholinergic deficiency state attributable to the underlying vascular dementia), avoidance of dopamine agonists (so as not to exacerbate dopamine-associated symptoms such as hallucinations), and avoidance of other possible delirium promoting agents such as benzodiazepines and opioids are the first elements of treatment. In terms of psychopharmacological interventions for delirium, antipsychotics are the best-established treatment; for avoidance of motor side effects, the atypical antipsychotics are increasingly popular. Because this will typically be a short-term use of atypical antipsychotics under close clinical surveillance, the risk of complications from the atypical antipsychotic agents themselves appears safely low, although the final word has not been written on this issue as yet.

Once the acute delirium is treated, continued reassessment for underlying vascular dementia and/or depression can proceed. If patients show persistent cognitive impairment when no longer showing specific signs of delirium, then cholinesterase inhibitors (although an off-label use) are increasingly considered state-of-the-art treatment for vascular dementia. These agents should be combined with continuing close clinical follow-up for assiduous management of the ongoing vascular disease by medical control of vascular risk factors.

Finally, the clinician must recognize that depression is quite common in vascular disease patients. Therefore, the clinical threshold to treat with antidepressants should be quite low. In antidepressant treatment of patients with systemic illnesses, it is helpful to pay particular attention to the issue of drug–drug interactions with selective serotonin reuptake inhibitors (SSRIs). For this reason, the usual SSRIs to recommend are escitalopram, citalopram, and lower dosages of sertraline; the agents fluoxetine, paroxetine, and fluvoxamine are all associated with drug–drug interactions and thus may be less safe in the patient with a complicated pharmacological regimen (Sandson et al. 2005).

QT$_c$ Prolongation and Atypical Antipsychotics

The patient was a 55-year-old white male admitted to the intensive care unit with altered mental status after a motor vehicle accident.

He had no formal psychiatric history. Computed tomography scans of the head were normal. Mental status examination revealed altered level of consciousness, decreased cognitive performance, and fluctuating mental status with intermittent visual hallucinations, including seeing "bugs and animals in my room." He was initially treated with haloperidol but experienced muscle dystonia. Thereafter, he was started on risperidone 1 mg twice a day and also received risperidone 0.5 mg twice daily as needed for agitation and delirium. His delirium symptoms improved, and his cognitive status returned to an unimpaired range, but 12-lead electrocardiography revealed that his QT_c interval had increased from a baseline 440 msec to 490 msec. Risperidone was discontinued, and he was subsequently treated with olanzapine 5 mg orally twice a day for several days before it was also discontinued. His QT_c interval returned to baseline. His delirium symptoms did not recur.

◆ **Diagnosis: Axis I—Delirium, 293.0; Adverse Effects of Medication Not Otherwise Specified, 995.2**

The atypical antipsychotics (risperidone, ziprasidone, olanzapine, quetiapine, aripiprazole, and clozapine) have revolutionized the treatment of psychotic illness. Increasingly, these agents have earned a place in the psychosomatic medicine armamentarium (Seitz et al. 2007). Beyond the logical choice for the in-hospital management of schizophrenia-spectrum disorders with concurrent medical-surgical illness, these agents are used for delirium and as nonspecific anxiolytics, sedatives, and hypnotic agents. The advantages over typical antipsychotics in terms of lower rates of anticholinergic and movement disorder side effects for these agents are generally appreciated by patients and physicians alike.

However, there is literature describing QT_c prolongation with atypical antipsychotics (Glassman and Bigger 2001). As such, due caution is advised when using these agents with cardiac patients, especially those with conduction system disease. In hospitalized patients, it is advisable to routinely obtain a pretreatment 12-lead electrocardiogram before treatment with atypical antipsychotic agents. One practice is to avoid risperidone, ziprasidone, and quetiapine if the baseline QT_c interval is greater than 450 msec and to monitor all cases when these three agents are used in patients with QT_c intervals less than 450 msec; such patients who subsequently significantly increase their QT_c (e.g., to over 500 msec) should then have risperidone, ziprasidone, or quetiapine discontinued.

In the patient with a baseline long QT_c who presents with a need for an antipsychotic agent, based on the current experience, it may be safer to consider olanzapine or aripiprazole. However, olanzapine is problematic in diabetic patients, and the clinical data on aripiprazole are at this point minimal for psychosomatic medicine uses of this medication. Psychosomatic medicine psychiatrists are well served by a practice pattern of routinely obtaining 12-lead electrocardiograms for patients in whom atypical antipsychotics are anticipated, especially in critically ill, intensive care unit, or cardiac patients.

Cardiac Effects of Overdose: Marital Issues and Body Image Issues

A 36-year-old lethargic female was brought to the emergency department by a friend who became concerned by the patient's slurred speech. The patient acknowledged drinking "quite a bit" of rum and taking approximately 100 mg of cyclobenzaprine because "I am tired of my mind racing; I just want to sleep." Frightened by what she had done, the patient had then called her friend on the telephone. Although drowsy, the patient denied any formal psychiatric history except episodic bingeing and purging over a 3-year period in college in her early 20s.

Her blood alcohol level was 251 mg/dL. A urine drug screening was positive only for cyclobenzaprine. There were no other active medical problems. When the patient was more alert, she described recent insomnia, a feeling that life was "dull and gray," ruminative doubts about her self-worth, diminished energy, making uncharacteristic mistakes at work, urges to binge, fantasizing about purging again, and two public tearful outbursts that had caught her by surprise. She denied suicidal ideation but dolefully said maybe her 7-year-old son's grandmother "would be a better parent" than she had been. Despite her initial complaint that her mind had been racing, further interview gave no evidence of a bipolar history or diathesis.

The patient reported that a contentious, prolonged divorce from her first husband had been finalized exactly 1 year earlier. Adding insult to injury, her younger sister, a part-time model, was married 2 weeks before the overdose. As a member of the wedding party, the patient had felt uncomfortably and persistently self-conscious at the wedding about having gained several pounds since the last family reunion. She was convinced, but not with delusional intensity, that her friends and family had noticed and critically commented on her weight gain. Eventually she acknowledged a few episodes of purging and obtaining an unidentified diuretic in the 2 weeks since the wedding. Two days before her presentation to the emergency department, the patient had discovered that the married man with whom she was having an affair was simultaneously cultivating yet another relationship.

◆ **Diagnosis: Axis I—Adjustment Disorder With Depressed Mood, 309.0; Rule Out Eating Disorder Not Otherwise Specified, 307.50**

This patient encountered converging biopsychosocial assaults. She had unwittingly set the stage for a potentially serious cardiac dysrhythmia with her use of a diuretic and her purging. Confounding this further, cyclobenzaprine has a tricyclic chemical structure that can precipitate torsades de pointes. A QRS of 0.12 msec warranted keeping the patient on a unit with electrocardiographic monitoring for 36 hours after admission until her QRS had returned to her baseline. The patient's long-standing struggles with body image were underscored by the anniversary of her divorce and the vivid perception that her weight gain was on display for all to see at the recent family wedding. This heightened sensitivity to appearance and anxiety about her physical desirability was seemingly confirmed and further aggravated when she learned that her current partner's devotion was illusory. After correction of her hypokalemia and normalization of her electrocardiogram, the patient accepted transfer to an inpatient psychiatric unit.

Methamphetamine Dependence and Cardiomyopathy

Methamphetamine abuse and dependence, which is approaching epidemic levels in various areas of the United States, is associated with many psychiatric and systemic complications. Notable among these are its cardiac effects, sometimes leading to severe cardiac impairment in young patients.

The patient was a 27-year-old single white male. He had begun the regular daily use of methamphetamine in his early teens. During periods of heavy use he would experience hallucinations while intoxicated; when withdrawing from methamphetamine, he would have

periods of several days of significantly depressed mood and profound fatigue. He would quickly return to methamphetamine use,
which was associated with improvement in his mood state. Thus was
established a pattern of perverse incentives.

Not surprisingly, he quickly developed numerous psychosocial
problems referable to his drug abuse. He could not maintain steady
employment, he was frequently homeless, and he served time in jail
and prison for possession and distribution of methamphetamine. He
had had a series of extremely dysfunctional and ultimately failed relationships with several substance-dependent women. He had no
close friends and he had recently been released from incarceration
yet another time for drug offenses. He was completely estranged
from his family, who had clearly "had enough" of his drug use and
his repeated and failed attempts to achieve and maintain sobriety.

He was seen in psychosomatic medicine consultation for "depression" when admitted to cardiology. He had developed chronic
fatigue, intolerance of physical exertion, and shortness of breath.
Cardiac evaluation including echocardiography revealed severe left
ventricular disease with an ejection fraction of less than 10%. On examination, he was an irritable, angry young man. He had a sense of
entitlement and grandiosity, with a tendency to blame others for his
suffering and to deny his own responsibility for his drug abuse and
resultant psychosocial and medical problems. He was only minimally able to process the seriousness of his heart disease.

He was treated with a low dosage of escitalopram for his mood
symptoms; this was well tolerated. He was eventually discharged to
a homeless shelter with a plan for medical and mental health follow-
up in the county system. He was advised to attend Narcotics Anonymous meetings and to obtain a sponsor in an effort to pursue recovery.

♦ **Diagnosis: Axis I—Amphetamine Dependence, 304.40;
Substance-Induced Mood Disorder, 292.84; Axis II—
Narcissistic Personality Disorder, 301.81**

Of all the systemic complications of methamphetamine dependence, end-stage cardiac disease may well be the most serious and
life threatening. Because of their substance dependence and, typically, their social isolation and lack of both medical compliance and
social support, these patients are poor candidates (from a psychosocial perspective) for heart transplantation. Their substance-induced
depressive disorder may be exacerbated by depression related to the
heart disease itself; in these patients, the depressed mood state is a

strong incentive to seek out a return to abuse of methamphetamine so as to self-medicate the mood state.

Clinical intervention by psychosomatic medicine physicians may be critical. Early treatment with a medically safe antidepressant is important for persistent depressive symptoms; it is usually impractical to wait several weeks after methamphetamine withdrawal for the mood state to rebound to a less depressed status. The frequent comorbidity of narcissistic personality disorder in these patients may be itself associated with irritability, particularly when the cardiac disease is interpreted as a narcissistic loss of the physical integrity of the self. It is clearly untenable to maintain a stance of physical grandiosity while simultaneously confronting severe functional impairment due to extremely limited cardiac output with associated symptoms of physical impairment.

Supportive psychotherapy and clear expectation of a commitment to a substance abuse recovery program is imperative; for those patients capable of adequate insight, psychotherapy approaches directed toward confrontation of physical impairment and threat to the integrity of the self can be attempted. If these patients can achieve substance abstinence and recovery, and can establish robust levels of social support and demonstrate medical compliance, they may then have their heart transplant candidacy reassessed.

Panic Disorder With Coronary Artery Disease: "A Chicken and an Egg"

Panic disorder is a common condition; because of its significantly "somatic" presentation, it often presents in a systemic general medical context rather than in a specialty psychiatric one. Psychosomatic medicine physicians will frequently encounter panic-spectrum symptoms in cardiac patients. Although it is appealing in some cases to consider panic disorder "versus" cardiac disease, many vexing cases will have significant elements of both. Importantly to the psychosomatic medicine physician, clinical intervention for the "psychiatric" aspects of the case may be relatively straightforward and may then help to sort out the differential aspects of the case.

> The patient was a 60-year-old divorced white female. Although she had had no formal psychiatric care ever before, she had a long period

of untreated and escalating panic attacks beginning in her 40s. She would develop spontaneous panic attacks with shortness of breath, choking, palpitations, and a feeling of "doom" that some unspecified disasters would befall her. She eventually limited her social behavior to where she would leave her home only for the most necessary activities. She lived simply and marginally for many years without treatment.

However, in her middle 50s, she developed coronary artery disease with angina. In addition, she developed cardiac valve disease and was admitted to the medical center for combined CABG and valve repair. Facing the threat to her health and survival, and anxious about being in a new and unfamiliar environment, she had an increase in the frequency and intensity of her panic attacks, leading to a psychosomatic medicine consultation. On examination, she was cognitively intact, mildly depressed, and notably anxious. She had no suicidal ideation and no psychotic symptoms. Her MMSE score was in the normal range.

She was treated with sertraline 50 mg daily and lorazepam 1 mg orally every 6 hours as needed for panic attacks. She tolerated the medication well and responded promptly to the as-needed lorazepam when taken. Her panic attacks in the hospital were much less frequent and disruptive, and her baseline level of anxiety decreased. She was thereafter able to proceed with cardiac surgery. She was kept on the psychotropic medications, and outpatient psychiatric follow-up was arranged.

◆ Diagnosis: Axis I—Panic Disorder With (Mild) Agoraphobia, 300.21

Panic disorder symptoms overlap significantly with those of angina; indeed, panic disorder is a common eventual diagnosis in the "recurrent atypical chest pain with a negative cardiac catheterization" patient. As such, psychosomatic medicine physicians should be particularly vigilant for panic disorder in the emergency presentation of chest pain that eventually is ruled out for cardiac disease. In this case, upon close examination, it was determined our patient had a long history of unmistakable panic disorder with mild agoraphobia. This patient, quite isolated socially, had experienced untreated panic disorder for 20 years.

When she later developed heart disease, the need for hospitalization and the sense of threat to her physical health were associated with increased anxiety and, not surprisingly, increased panic attacks.

Fortunately, she had a robust response to routine treatment with psychotropic medication for panic disorder and was thereafter able to better tolerate the hospitalization and cardiac surgery. The "synergy" of panic disorder and concurrent cardiac disease should be considered when both illnesses present simultaneously or, as in this case, sequentially. Intervention for panic disorder may result in the patient being better able to tolerate needed treatment for cardiac disease.

Self-Inflicted Stab Wound to the Heart

Occasionally patients will injure themselves in the heart in the context of suicidal behavior. If the patient then suffers functional impairment to the heart, functional adaptation to new limitations in cardiac status may be additively difficult for patients already experiencing poor coping responses to external stressors.

> The patient was a 28-year-old single white male with no prior history of psychiatric illness. He had been accused of theft in his workplace, which he vehemently denied. However, as law enforcement investigation became more intrusive to him, he began to develop paranoid delusions of various others being "out to get" him. This expanded to include people who had no plausible connection to the alleged theft of property. He began to experience insomnia and anxiety in addition to his paranoid delusions.
>
> At the culmination of these symptoms, he became convinced that it would be better to kill himself rather than suffer some worse fate at the hands of his imagined antagonists. In a suicide attempt, he stabbed himself in the middle of the chest with an ice pick. The tool entered his pericardium and penetrated both ventricles. Immediately after stabbing himself, he suddenly realized the gravity of what he had done and called for assistance. He was taken to the emergency department with the ice pick still in his chest and was admitted; the ice pick was carefully removed without surgical complications. However, functional assessment with echocardiography revealed him to have a postoperative ejection fraction of only 30% (presumably, immediately prior to the wound he had been normal).
>
> After he was stabilized and in need of no further surgery, he was then transferred to psychiatry. Curiously, he no longer endorsed the extreme anxiety and the paranoia that he had been experiencing before injuring himself. It almost seemed that the self-harm act had somehow "relieved" him of the psychotic thought processes that had been bedeviling him. He was able to verbalize understanding of

the nature of his cardiac injury and his new functional impairment, and he agreed to continued follow-up with cardiology. He was not treated with antipsychotic medications, and he was eventually discharged in stable condition.

♦ **Diagnosis: Axis I—Brief Psychotic Disorder, 298.8**

This patient had become psychotic over a relatively short period of time, in the context of severe stressors of having been accused of a crime. His paranoid delusions and associated anxiety increased to the point where a serious suicide attempt was made because he could not bear to further tolerate his paranoid delusions. He punctured both ventricles. Immediately, he felt remorse for his act and he then sought out medical treatment appropriately. Curiously, when evaluated after the stab wound, he was no longer psychotic. It was almost as if his self-inflicted wound represented an act of atonement for a perceived transgression or shortcoming. In individual psychotherapy sessions, he was enormously regretful of his self-stabbing. He was aware of the physiological consequences of his injury to the heart and agreed to be compliant with follow-up cardiology care. As he had reconstituted his baseline level of function following a symptomatic period of less than 30 days, he met diagnostic criteria for brief psychotic disorder.

References

Burns A, Gallagley A, Byrne J: Delirium. J Neurol Neurosurg Psychiatry 75:362–367, 2004

Folstein MF, Folstein SE, McHugh PR: "Mini-Mental State": a practical method for grading the cognitive state of patients for the clinician. J Psychiatr Res 12:189–198, 1975

Glassman AH, Bigger JT: Antipsychotic drugs: prolonged QT_c interval, torsades de pointes, and sudden death. Am J Psychiatry 158:1774–1782, 2001

Litaker D, Locala J, Franco K, et al: Preoperative risk factors for postoperative delirium. Gen Hosp Psychiatry 23:84–89, 2001

Sandson NB, Armstrong SC, Cozza KL: An overview of psychotropic drug–drug interactions. Psychosomatics 46:464–494, 2005

Seitz DP, Gill SS, van Zyl LT: Antipsychotics in the treatment of delirium: a systematic review. J Clin Psychiatry 68:11–21, 2007

4

LUNG DISEASE

Pulmonary disease in all of its manifestations (respiratory distress, hypoxic injury to the central nervous system, and cases with delirium associated with respiratory compromise) make up a significant part of the clinical caseload of an inpatient psychosomatic medicine service. Even when patients are discharged to outpatient care, their tenuous pulmonary status may keep them in a state of anxious distress. Acute pulmonary compromise can lead to terrifying symptoms of suffocation that can resemble panic attacks. Prolonged intubation and ventilation is commonly associated with delirium; the eventual weaning of ventilatory support may be limited by significant anxiety symptoms. For the occasional patient, the extreme intervention of lung transplantation may represent the best chance at survival or a higher quality of function. Thus, pulmonary disease patients are of particular interest to psychosomatic medicine psychiatrists.

Severe Asthma, Disability, and Depression

The patient was a 50-year-old divorced white female. She had no significant medical or psychiatric history; notably, she had never been a smoker. She had been raised in a dysfunctional home by a harsh, demanding, and highly critical father and a submissive, dependent, acquiescent, yet quietly hostile mother. She developed an avoidant and obsessive-compulsive character style where she was very demanding of her own performance, blamed herself for all her difficulties, and was unable to ask for help even when she was in great need. She had been married once and was divorced. She was never able to sustain an intimate relationship with a man for more than 4 years; she would describe herself as "always picking the

wrong men," with numerous issues such as drug abuse, physical assaultiveness, or anger management problems.

Approximately 15 years earlier, the patient had had insidious
onset of episodic shortness of breath and was diagnosed with adult-
onset asthma. Unfortunately, despite aggressive medical management, her asthma progressed, and she had severe functional impairment by age 45. She was oxygen dependent at night, required
breathing treatments with nebulized bronchodilators every 2 hours,
and was steroid dependent. As her functional status deteriorated,
she became unable to work and was placed on disability retirement.
She developed episodes of irritability and depression that became
worse as she became steroid dependent and experienced physical
impairment and loss of income.

She was referred for psychiatric care by her long-time pulmonologist, who was concerned about her increasing depression. Psychopharmacological treatment with duloxetine and quetiapine
significantly improved her mood, but she remained very vulnerable
to mood exacerbations when difficulties arose in her family (her father developed dementia and needed to be institutionalized; at the
same time, her mother developed progressively critical chronic obstructive pulmonary disorder and died) and when her pulmonary
disease worsened. These mood exacerbations were also notable
when her daily dosage of prednisone exceeded 40 mg, as was frequently necessary.

After the death of her mother and the continued debility of her father, she and her male partner of 2½ years separated. Her partner
had become increasingly impatient in tolerating the physical limitations associated with her pulmonary illness and withdrew any emotional support. She was able, through psychotherapy, to see how her
father's critical and self-centered nature was repeatedly recapitulated
in her relationship with other men. During this time her pulmonary
status continued to deteriorate, with persistent CO_2 retention and
diaphragmatic flattening.

She was then referred by her pulmonologist for an evaluation for
double lung transplant. She was understandably frightened at the
prospect of an extremely long operation with significant risks for
operative mortality and was also self-conscious about having large
postoperative scars. Nonetheless, she was willing to undergo the
transplant operation. To qualify for the operation, she was required
to develop a postoperative plan whereby she would relocate to Los
Angeles (the site of the transplant operation) for a 6-week period of
postoperative monitoring, which would require a family member to
be present 24 hours a day. She was initially very hesitant to approach
her family members (including her daughter) to ask for this assis-

tance. She was finally able to do so when it became clear that without such a family care plan, she would not be considered for the surgery.

◆ **Diagnosis: Axis I—Major Depression, Recurrent, Severe Without Psychotic Features, 296.33**

This patient's long-standing and intermittent depression can be understood well in psychodynamic terms. She was the child of a hypercritical, sarcastic, and judgmental father and a quiet and dependent yet hostile mother. Her father's constant criticism and making fun of her physical appearance and other attributes led to a poor core sense of self. Her relationships with men were characterized by brief attachments to men who were typically self-centered, irritable, and angry "just like my father." Nonetheless, she was able to function reasonably well in business and as a single parent until the development of severe asthma. The loss of her self-perception as a healthy person was very difficult for her. She could no longer work in business, an important source of mastery and independence.

Once she was on a regular medication regimen for her lung disease, she became sensitive to psychiatric side effects from her medications. She would get notably more depressed when her steroid dosage was increased to treat exacerbations of pulmonary failure; she was able to accurately self-observe these emotional symptoms, and they would improve somewhat when the steroid dosage was returned back to maintenance levels.

Another aspect of this case was what the patient would call a "silent disability." Because the severe asthma was not disfiguring, she said that others did not easily understand her as ill. Because her pulmonary illness was "just asthma," she would meet others who would view this as a somewhat "trivial" illness and not a valid explanation for her major functional impairment. Others would disapprove of her use of a "handicapped" vehicle pass and preferential parking, even though she was unable to walk even modest distances without needing extra breathing treatments.

When offered the chance at a double lung transplant, she was of mixed feelings. Hopeful that the operation would rescue her from a life of otherwise stultifying dependence on her pulmonary treatments, with an anticipated significant increase in physical endurance, she was nonetheless frightened of the serious operation and hesitant to turn to family members as helpful figures during the period of postsurgical recovery.

This case, although less dramatic than many, illustrates several points. There was an intimate connection between the status of her pulmonary and functional status and her degree of mood symptoms. Her mood symptoms were prone to steroid dosage–induced exacerbations. Her suffering with an illness that was not fully appreciated by others and trivialized by some as "only asthma" led to poor access to emotional support. Finally, she had to confront major morbidity and mortality in middle age while dealing with the death of her mother and the clinical decline of her father. This case illustrates how the psychotherapeutic approach to patients with chronic severe illness is well served by integrating psychodynamic and psychosomatic approaches.

Carbon Monoxide Poisoning and Hippocampal Necrosis

The patient was a 25-year-old single white male who was admitted for hyperbaric oxygen treatment following a suicide attempt. He had been depressed over the loss of a relationship with a young woman. He had rerouted the exhaust system of his car to discharge into the passenger compartment in a remote, isolated location. When found, he was emergently brought for hyperbaric oxygen treatment. Several hours after the hyperbaric treatment was completed, psychosomatic medicine evaluation was requested to "evaluate depression with a suicide attempt and rule out continued suicidality."

On examination, the patient's affect was curiously bright and pleasant, not at all "depressed." He denied any recent loss of a relationship; in fact, he did not even recall the name of the young woman in question. He said that no, he had not made a suicide attempt, and in fact had never been suicidal, asking "why would I be suicidal?"

His cognitive examination, however, was ominous. He claimed the year was "1990" (factually 1995) and that he was "20" (not 25, his actual age) years old. All of his recall of his personal history stopped as though "frozen in time" 5 years before. He was not depressed over losing the relationship, because he did not recall ever having had it. His recall memory was impaired, as was his orientation; other aspects of the mental status examination were normal.

Magnetic resonance imaging scans showed bilateral hippocampal necrosis. When reinterviewed the next day, he said he was pleased to meet the examiner, whom he claimed to never have met before. The balance of his examination was unchanged from that of the previous day. This man had a remarkably "pure" amnestic disorder from bilateral hippocampal lesions; this was not dementia related, because other cognitive functions were preserved. He was transferred to a rehabilitation facility.

♦ **Diagnosis: Axis I—Amnestic Disorder Due to Carbon Monoxide Poisoning, 294.0; Adjustment Disorder With Depressed Mood, 309.0**

One relatively infrequently encounters "pure" amnestic disorders in clinical practice; the majority of patients with clinically significant amnesia either have either "static to progressive" cognitive deficits and thus qualify for a diagnosis of dementia or have the spectrum of cognitive and circadian/behavioral disturbances that are classified as delirium. Numerous aspects were striking about this case. The patient had been significantly depressed over the loss of a relationship; although, importantly, by the time he was interviewed he had no memory of the relationship, its denouement, or his period of depressed mood leading to his (also not recalled) suicidal ideation and suicide attempt. Therefore, in the absence of clear and convincing collateral history of a major mood disorder (his family members were shocked to discover his suicide attempt because he had left few clues as to his psychic suffering), a retrospective diagnosis of a depressive episode versus adjustment disorder was somewhat speculative.

Indeed, when questioned about his mood state, he responded with a sense of puzzlement, because he had "nothing to be depressed about." This was itself remarkable, because suicide attempt survivors with mood disorders often have strong emotional reactions (e.g., guilt, remorse, profound relief over survival, or continued suicidality with an intention of "getting it right next time") upon physical recovery from the medical consequences of the attempt.

On formal cognitive examination, he was remarkably unimpaired in other spheres of cognitive activity, aside from profound amnesia. In light of the absence of dementia affecting multiple spheres of cognitive function and given his preserved sociability and (now) unremarkable affective state, it would have been possible to minimize his deficits. The encounter with this man had the flavor of film and literary portrayals of parodies of amnestic states with continual reliving of events. The focal nature of his amnesia (without dementia) was substantiated in the magnetic resonance imaging findings of isolated bilateral hippocampal necrosis.

The impact on his very supportive extended family was profound. They had experienced a remarkable "roller coaster" of emotional reactions to his case. They were initially devastated at the discovery of his suicide attempt, then anxiously apprehensive during his emergent transport to the hyperbaric oxygen unit, and then extraordinarily grateful for access to the probable life-saving treatment of hyperbaric oxygen, only to finally come to terms with the profundity of cognitive impairment resulting from his new-onset amnestic disorder. The patient was, of course, unable to learn of his predicament and remained somewhat oblivious to and puzzled by the events around, and about, him.

Psychosomatic medicine physicians treating survivors of carbon monoxide poisoning (either intentional or accidental), including those physicians consulting to medical centers with hyperbaric oxygen treatment units, should keep such diagnoses in mind when confronting this particular clinical circumstance. Neuroimaging specifically examining the hippocampal structures may reveal lesions corresponding to isolated amnestic disorders.

Echolalia and Hypoxia

The patient was a 65-year-old white male with chronic obstructive pulmonary disorder and oxygen dependence. He was admitted to the medical center with acute mental status changes. He had no prior history of psychiatric illness or treatment. The history of present illness (which was obtained from family members) was that he had been in his usual status of tenuous but otherwise stable physical health until the day before. His family had suspected that he had self-discontinued his home oxygen in order to smoke; this was a familiar pattern for him. He had been warned of the dangers of smoking while the oxygen was running and had told his primary care physician that he would "promise to turn the oxygen off if I have a cigarette."

When he was admitted to the hospital, he exhibited extremely regressed mental status. Although he was alert and not physically agitated, he had no spontaneous speech. He would not answer examiner questions but would rather "parrot" the examiner's words back to him verbatim; this represented the relatively rare symptom of echolalia.

His oxygen was restarted, and he was observed closely in the hospital overnight. The next day, he had completely recovered his cognitive function. His examination was now unremarkable. He was now able confirm that, yes, he had "snuck" a cigarette but that he had "been careful" to turn off his oxygen before smoking it "because I promised my doctor I wouldn't smoke with the oxygen on." He had absolutely no memory of the events between the smoking of the cigarette and then coming into consciousness in the hospital, a period of 1–2 days.

◆ **Diagnosis: Axis I—Delirium, 293.0**

In terms of explaining this case, the formulation derived was that the patient was chronically so tenuously compensated with his pulmonary status that even the brief loss of supplemental oxygen was enough to decompensate his cognitive function to isolated echolalia, which was completely reversed once supplemental oxygen was resumed. Patients with severely compromised pulmonary function may present with acute delirium at any time if their pulmonary status is altered, such as from a temporary interruption of the supply of supplemental oxygen as in this case. Close monitoring of mental status (including cognitive status) and arterial blood gases and/or pulse oximetry readings may allow for correlations between pulmonary status and mental status. When such patients require pharmacological treatment, agents with a possible association with decreased respiratory drive (e.g., benzodiazepines) should be avoided so as not to compromise an already tenuous respiratory status.

Cystic Fibrosis and Psychopathology

Occasionally encountered in adult psychosomatic medicine, cystic fibrosis is an example of a chronic illness associated with significantly shortened life expectancy and much functional impairment as well as the likelihood of episodic decompensation and hospitalizations for gastrointestinal and pulmonary complications. Because it usually presents in childhood, the patient often early on identifies him- or herself as chronically ill, dependent, and vulnerable. Yet these patients do not necessarily appear grossly impaired to others, who thus may not empathically understand the loss of function and degree of impairment and threat to physical integrity with which these patients live.

Case 1

The patient was a 19-year-old single white female with a history of cystic fibrosis since early childhood. She had had chronic poor gastrointestinal and pulmonary function with resulting wasting, fatigue, and poor exercise tolerance. She had largely been abandoned by peers, who progressed through normative social, educational, and employment stages of development, leaving her behind.

She was grateful for her high level of support from her family and physicians yet resented her disability and yearned to be "normal" in ways she knew were not possible. She had developed chronic depression in the context of her physical illness and its associated psychosocial losses. She was able to discuss how only a lung transplant operation would give her any reasonable hope for improved and stable pulmonary function.

♦ **Diagnosis: Axis I—Major Depressive Disorder, Single Episode, Moderate (Chronic), 296.22**

Case 2

The patient was a 23-year-old white female who had had a particularly difficult course of cystic fibrosis. She was the only child of very supportive parents. As a young teenager, she developed cystic fibrosis–related liver failure and received a liver transplant. She subsequently did relatively well for several years but later developed a more malignant course with her pulmonary disease. She had frequent hospitalizations for acute respiratory distress requiring treatment with antibiotics.

She was briefly able to move into her own apartment at age 21. (Her parents continued to fully support her financially because she was unable to maintain employment.) The independence this move symbolized was very important to her, as was her ability to self-manage her many medical appointments, laboratory tests, and medications. Unfortunately, due to her recurrent pulmonary disease, she was unable to climb the steps at the apartment and had to return to her parents' home. Although her parents were respectful of whatever independence she could manage and were supportive at all times, the return home was a major narcissistic injury to her. She became depressed (with a notable fatigue component) in the context of dealing with her illness and was treated successfully with bupropion 150 mg daily.

Because of chronic gastrointestinal compromise from her cystic fibrosis, she was chronically cachectic with marginal nutritional status. As her lung disease progressed, it became evident that she might become a candidate for lung transplantation to improve her pulmonary status. However, because of her marginal nutritional status, she was not a surgical candidate until she improved her nutrition.

In psychotherapy sessions, this patient was able to quite realistically look at her severe illness and the likelihood of a very limited life expectancy (even if she were to receive a lung transplant operation) and was able to discuss age-normative struggles for a degree of social independence from her family, all the while being appreciative of their ongoing and strong social support. She longed for even modest normative experiences of independence, work, and social relationships. Notable in this woman was a complete lack of self-pity or resentment of her illness and what it had cost her. She quite admirably maintained a stance of trying to remain optimistic yet simultaneously realistic.

◆ **Diagnosis: Axis I—Depressive Disorder Not Otherwise Specified, 311**

Cystic fibrosis as illustrated in this case is a model of the young adult survivor of a pediatric onset chronic illness. Other ready examples are systemic lupus erythematosus and diabetes mellitus. The chronicity of illness robs the patient of normative experiences of childhood and the adolescent "omnipotence" and grandiosity that most young adults go through before settling on their adult identity. When one is ill, particularly with a chronic, relapsing, and life-threatening illness, such an age-normative sense of omnipotence is irreconcilable with the facts of the illness. The illness may thus be expected to significantly color and limit the worldview of this chronically ill young adult.

Some affected patients may seek escapism through acting-out behaviors such as substance abuse, with its predictable painful consequences. Others may develop depression, psychodynamically rooted in the irreconcilable differences between age-appropriate omnipotence, grandiosity, and experimentation with social roles and the numerous limitations imposed by the chronic illness. The psychotherapy approach to these patients may include empathic confrontation of the irony of this dilemma.

Persistence of dependency (in these cases, the dependency object being the medical care system) can be a striking part of these patients' experience; they may need permission to express anger for the injustice of their situations, but the psychotherapist can empathically direct the patients' rage toward the illness itself rather than toward their caretakers and medical personnel, upon whom the patient remains (of course) profoundly dependent.

GASTROINTESTINAL DISORDERS

The brain/mind and the gut are often connected in clinical practice. Beyond the obvious connections between psychosomatic medicine psychiatry and the hospitalized eating disorder patient, the areas of brain/gut interaction include depression with appetite disturbance, behavioral complications of gastric bypass procedures, psychotic delusions of gastrointestinal illness, and conditions such as irritable bowel syndrome that are often experienced by clinicians as having a significant behavioral component. Additionally, there is the psychiatric suffering associated with complicated and disfiguring major gastrointestinal surgical procedures, dependency on total parenteral nutrition and other parenteral supports for impaired gastrointestinal function, and the existential threat represented by gastrointestinal cancers. Liver disease is a common complication of substance abuse, and treatment of liver disease is itself associated with psychiatric side effects. Therefore, the gastrointestinal system is a common site of illnesses associated with significant degrees of psychopathology. Complicating psychosomatic medicine management in many cases is the fact that nearly all psychotropic agents are only available in oral form, dramatically limiting psychopharmacological options for intervention.

Demoralization and Multiple Medical Problems in a Gastrointestinal Surgery Case

A walk from the parking lot to the emergency department may be the start of an arduous journey. The course of a hospital stay may include unexpected switchbacks, valleys and steep ascents. A 54-year-old male convenience mart owner with long-standing chronic obstructive pulmonary disease, diabetes mellitus type II, hypertension, paroxysmal atrial fibrillation, peripheral vascular disease, and morbid obesity presented with acute abdominal pain leading to discovery of a perforated duodenal ulcer. He underwent an antrectomy and Billroth II reconstruction.

Despite prophylactic anticoagulation, the patient developed a popliteal artery thrombosis while recuperating from the abdominal surgery. His right lower extremity became irreversibly ischemic, and he was obliged to accept a below-the-knee amputation of his right leg. The patient's peripheral vascular disease, diabetic vasculopathy, and obesity conspired to impede healing of the stump wound, and he experienced recurrent wound dehiscence. Each episode necessitated yet another debridement, and polymicrobial infections of the wound were common complications. The medical and surgical teams were not surprised by the onset of a *Clostridium difficile* superinfection, but it was an unforeseen and frustrating development for the patient. Not long after resolution of his associated diarrhea, he developed the characteristic pain and cutaneous blisters of herpes zoster. He was treated with acyclovir and transdermal fentanyl.

The patient's wife had initially doubled her time at the convenience mart to cover her husband's work hours but now felt torn between the need to visit him in the hospital and the need to sustain their business. Meanwhile, the patient felt bereft of autonomy in multiple spheres, isolated by recurring infectious disease precautions procedures, being manifestly unproductive, burdened by mounting bills, and uncertain when he could dare hope to be released from hospital. He developed persistent atrial fibrillation and was eventually treated with an anticoagulant, warfarin. On the day prior to the request for a psychiatric consultation to assess for depression, the patient developed gross hematuria despite a therapeutic international normalized ratio of 2.3.

Although the patient described discouragement and fatigue, he did not feel utterly hopeless and was not willing to endorse that each day felt like a "burden on his back." His sleep had become fragmented and his appetite was diminished, but he was more bothered by the nagging perception that he was letting his wife down and failing to protect her from having to work too hard at the store. He described the modest goal of a viable small, independent business and a cabin on a nearby lake that he and his wife had embraced years before. It had seemed as though the whole of his past had equipped him with the skills and wherewithal to see this venture through to successful completion. As a couple they had begun to talk of selling the convenience mart in 10 years and moving to live at the lake year-round. However, the patient's nearly 5 months in hospital had ruptured the sense of continuity between past effort and future rewards. He felt bewildered and uncertain but declined to endorse depression per se. Explaining some of what he had experienced, such as the clostridial infection and the rationale for anticoagulation with atrial fibrillation, seemed to buoy his spirits.

◆ **Diagnosis: Axis I—Phase of Life Problem, V62.89; Rule Out Adjustment Disorder Unspecified, 309.9**

Symptoms of demoralization may overlap with those of major depression. The diagnostic waters may be further clouded in patients with extensive medical/surgical debilitation who understandably encounter collateral vegetative difficulties with sleep, energy, and appetite. The distinction is worth pursuing because demoralization can be actively addressed at the bedside. A psychotherapeutic relationship, however brief, that reminds the patient that his distress "makes sense" can enable the patient to put his suffering in perspective and recapture a sense of hope and purpose in living.

Drs. James Griffith and Lynne Gaby (2005) suggested that the consultation psychiatrist is well positioned to help the patient shift his existential perspective from a state of vulnerability to a "posture of resilience." They noted that each existential state cited can be displaced by a corresponding perspective that infuses resilience—that is, trust rather than fear, communion rather than isolation, coherence rather than confusion, hope rather than despair, a sense of agency rather than helplessness, purpose rather than meaninglessness, and joy rather than sorrow.

Griffith and Gaby offer examples of questions that help a patient reflect on his or her life's experience and potentially move from an existential position of vulnerability to a posture of resilience. Each consultation psychiatrist can absorb these questions and find his or her own voice and style for supportively evoking the patient's recollection of people and events from the past that reinforce the will to persevere through difficult conditions.

Trust Versus Fear
- Who has given you a shoulder to lean on?
- Who relies on you? How did he/she first decide to trust you?
- [If religious] Does God keep his promises? How do you know?

Agency Versus Helplessness

+ What should I know about you as a person, beyond your illness?
+ What most helps you to stand strong against the challenges of this illness?
+ What are some steps you have taken to keep this illness from taking complete and total charge of your life?

Communion Versus Isolation

+ Who really understands your situation?
+ When you have difficult days, with whom do you talk?
+ In whose presence do you feel a bodily sense of peace?
+ [If religious] What does God know about your experience that other people do not understand?

Coherence Versus Confusion

+ How do you make sense of what you are going through?
+ When you are uncertain how to make sense of it, how do you deal with moments of feeling confused?
+ To whom do you turn when you feel confused?
+ [If religious] Do you sense that God sees any purpose in your suffering?

Purpose Versus Meaninglessness

+ What keeps you going on difficult days?
+ For whom, or for what, does it matter that you continue to live?
+ What do you hope to contribute with your life in the time you have remaining?
+ [If religious] What does God hope you will do with your life in days to come?

Hope Versus Despair

+ From what sources do you draw hope?
+ On difficult days, what keeps you from giving up?
+ Who have you known in your life who would not be surprised to see you hopeful amid adversity? What did this person know about you that other people may not have known?
+ *And if the patient replies, "But I have no hope…":* Was there a time when you did feel hope? How long has it been? What happened?

- If you were not so ill, do you suppose there would be things you would notice as signs of hope?
- As I hear your words and see your situation, what do you sense that I might consider to be a possible sign of hope?
- [If religious] Do you sense that God carries hope for your life? How so?

Joy Versus Sorrow

- What sustains your capacity to experience joy in the midst of pain?
- If you could look back upon this experience of illness from some future time, what would you say that you took from it that added to your life?

Acetaminophen Overdose and Death by Fulminant Liver Failure

A 42-year-old woman fought repeatedly with her husband over his unwillingness to help with basic housework. One evening, after they fought yet again over his refusal to help her with the dishes, he stormed out of the house. She became so angry that she impulsively took 50 extra-strength acetaminophen tablets, a total of 25 grams. When nothing immediately happened after the overdose, she went to bed, embarrassed by what she had done and determined to "sleep it off."

She awakened in the early morning hours nauseated and vomiting and continued to be intermittently ill throughout the night. Her husband had by then returned home and apologized to her, but she did not tell him about the overdose, continuing to feel foolish for having allowed herself to take pills over a marital spat. The next day, she at first refused to see a doctor, but as she persisted with her vomiting, her husband insisted on taking her to see their family physician.

Late in the afternoon, nearly 24 hours after the ingestion, after first denying that she had overdosed, she finally admitted to the doctor what she had done, and she was sent to the hospital emergency department for further evaluation and possible admission. After her transaminases were found to be in the 10,000 range, she was admitted to the intensive care unit and started on *N*-acetylcysteine therapy.

The next day, a psychiatry consult was placed. The psychiatrist found an alert, cooperative woman, euthymic without evidence for either psychosis or manic behavior, who described her shame at having risked her life over such a petty matter as her husband's resistance to helping with the dishes. The patient said that she did not know what had come over her, because she had never before—even in her teen years—made anything even remotely resembling a suicide attempt. She detailed how she and her husband had never managed conflict well in their 18-year marriage, and she expressed her ongoing resentment at what she perceived as the unequal division of labor in their home. She said that she had never seen a psychiatrist or therapist before, but she readily agreed with the consultant's recommendation for family therapy. She volunteered the suggestion that one of the pastors at her family's church was also a counselor and might be willing to provide that service.

As the psychiatrist was taking his leave of the patient, who had no other evident psychopathology than a partner-relational problem, the intensivist entered the room with the unwelcome news that her international normalized ratio had bumped to 4.1. He informed the patient that she would be imminently transferred to the medical center's transplant unit for observation in the context of acute liver failure and potential need for liver transplantation. Over the next 48 hours, the patient's toxic hepatitis continued to worsen. Disseminated intravascular coagulation ensued, and she required intubation and maximal life support. Before a donor liver could be located for emergent transplantation, she succumbed to fulminant hepatic failure.

◆ **Diagnosis: Axis I—Partner Relational Problem, V61.10; Delirium, 293.0**

This case graphically reminds the physician that death by overdose is not always intentional but can result from miscalculation, naïve notions that over-the-counter medications must be "safe" because they are readily available, or other distortions. The irony here is that this patient, save for the relational difficulties in her marriage, appeared to be free of mental illness before her fulminant liver failure. Had a donor liver been procured, the psychosomatic medicine psychiatrist would likely have had to make a decision on the suitability of the patient for transplant. When patients present in fulminant hepatic failure such as in this case, there is not the usual time for the patient and the family to gradually accept the expectations of liver transplantation, because the decision must be made emergently.

Gastric Bypass, Depression, and Borderline and Histrionic Personality Traits

Gastric bypass surgery for the treatment of extreme, life-threatening obesity is a more commonly performed surgery in recent years. With the contemporary epidemic of obesity in many populations, the likelihood is that this procedure will be even more commonly performed in the future. The psychosomatic medical management of these cases (both in terms of preoperative evaluation and postoperative management) is an important part of the psychosomatic service mission.

> The patient was a 52-year-old African American woman admitted to the gastrointestinal surgery service with dehydration and malnutrition following a gastric bypass surgery 4 months previously. The surgery team called for a psychosomatic medicine psychiatric consultation, suspecting an eating disorder, depression, and suicidal ideation in the patient.
>
> Upon evaluation, the patient noted that she vomited involuntarily "about 80% of the time" and "because I'm scared of gaining weight about 20% of the time." She had lost 100 pounds since her bypass surgery. Despite this apparent surgical success, she had felt "overwhelmed and discouraged" since her surgery. She was at risk of losing her part-time teaching job, her health insurance, and her home due to her many days of absence due to illness. She felt inadequately socially supported by her family, although she had four physician siblings and four adult children living in the local area. The patient believed that she had always been the "least successful" sibling and, as such, was embarrassed and thus reluctant to turn to her family for much financial and/or emotional support. The patient denied a history of psychiatric symptoms or treatment prior to the gastric bypass procedure and had been psychiatrically cleared by a psychosomatic medicine psychiatrist prior to the surgery.
>
> At the time of the evaluation, the patient was packing her bags and threatening to leave the hospital against medical advice. She reported feeling that she "should be able to handle the stress" of her circumstances by herself. She admitted to frequent thoughts of overdosing on insulin to commit suicide. She was motorically restless, tearful, and dysphoric. The psychosomatic medicine team prescribed sertraline and placed the patient on an involuntary psychiatric hold; she was then transferred to a separately located inpatient psychiatric facility for treatment of her mood disorder.
>
> The patient spent several days at an inpatient psychiatric treatment facility but soon returned to the university medical center for

treatment of hypoglycemia following an overdose on another patient's insulin. Notes from the psychiatric hospital staff described the patient's behavior as manipulative and disruptive. She was eventually medically stabilized after the insulin overdose and was returned to the inpatient psychiatric facility.

◆ **Diagnosis: Axis I—Depressive Disorder Not Otherwise Specified, 311; Eating Disorder Not Otherwise Specified, 307.50; Axis II—Borderline and Histrionic Traits**

Many medical centers performing gastric bypass surgery for obesity are now incorporating psychiatric evaluations into their preoperative evaluations. These evaluations are considered important for a number of reasons. Researchers have identified high rates of psychopathology in morbidly obese patients presenting for bariatric surgery (Sarwer et al. 2004). Higher rates of bulimia nervosa, mood disorders, anxiety disorders, and personality disorders have been found in weight loss surgery patients (Black et al. 1992; Grothe et al. 2006). Additionally, obesity is in part a behavioral disorder, and assessments of patients' ability to change their behavior and comply with rigid postoperative instructions and expectations can be useful in postoperative treatment planning (Grothe et al. 2006).

The Boston Interview has been constructed as a standardized interview tool for patients being evaluated for gastric bypass, with the expectation that data gathered will be useful for future research. The major areas covered by this assessment are 1) weight, diet, and nutrition history; 2) current eating behaviors; 3) medical history; 4) understanding of surgical procedures, risks, and the postsurgical regimen; 5) motivation and expectations of surgical outcome; 6) relationships and support system; and 7) psychiatric functioning (Sogg and Mor 2004).

Although the findings regarding psychopathology and postoperative weight loss outcome have generally shown no association, it appears that a history of psychiatric treatment prior to surgery may actually be associated with increased weight loss following surgery. The weight loss outcomes in patients with severe psychiatric problems preoperatively remain largely undefined, because many of these patients are excluded from surgery (Clark et al. 2003; Grothe et al. 2006).

In a systematic review of psychological and psychosocial predictors of weight loss and mental health after bariatric surgery, Herpertz et al. (2004) found that although preoperative psychiatric illness, including personality pathology, did not predict differences in postoperative weight loss, it was associated with psychiatric problems postoperatively. Patients undergoing weight loss surgery who have been sexually abused have shown increased rates of postoperative psychiatric hospitalization, although there was no relationship found between a history of sexual abuse and percentage of excess weight loss 2 years postoperatively (Clark et al. 2007).

A history of binge eating disorder preoperatively has been identified as a factor inhibiting postoperative weight loss in retrospective studies, but this finding has not been supported in prospective studies (Grothe et al. 2006; Hsu et al. 1998; Powers et al. 1999). The development of a new-onset eating disorder with features of both anorexia and bulimia, but not meeting full criteria for either disorder, has also been noted in post–gastric bypass patients (Segal et al. 2004). Segal et al. (2004) proposed criteria for "postsurgical eating avoidance disorder" based on a pattern emerging in some post-bypass patients.

The patient described in this case was evaluated by a psychosomatic medicine psychiatrist preoperatively, using a standardized interview that is similar to The Boston Interview for Gastric Bypass (Sogg and Mor 2004). The preoperative psychiatric evaluation included a full psychiatric history with particular attention paid to history of eating disorders, substance abuse, and sexual abuse; Axis I and Axis II psychopathology; social support; and weight loss expectations. Based on the preoperative evaluation, the patient was considered to be a low risk candidate. She appeared to be well informed about the surgery; she denied a history of binge eating, purging, anorexia, mood or anxiety disorder, substance abuse, or sexual abuse. She reported her social support network as strong.

The extent of this patient's postoperative psychopathology, including mood instability, purging behavior, and suicidality did not appear to have been predicted by her encouraging preoperative evaluation. Although it is possible that the patient did have a history of mood symptoms, interpersonal problems, or binge eating that she minimized in order to qualify for surgery, other contributors to her decompensation may have included the physical stress of surgery, the unexpected threatened loss of job and thus medical insurance as a result of frequent hospitalizations, and changes in her interpersonal relationships resulting from her weight loss. The presence of these factors and the reduction in availability of a major prior coping mechanism—eating—may have brought the patient to the point that she was no longer capable of regulating her affect and, in effect, regressed to very primitive defenses of splitting and projection.

Although the psychological outcomes in the 1–2 years following weight loss surgery appear generally positive, there continue to be reports of patients who experience psychiatric "side effects" of surgery including new substance abuse, suicidality, and impulsive behaviors (Grothe et al. 2006; Hsu et al. 1998; Sarwer et al. 2005). Hsu et al. (1998) suggested that future work with patients might include social skills training to help patients adjust to the psychosocial consequences of weight loss.

Gastric Bypass and Bipolar Disorder: Alternative Psychopharmacology

Gastric bypass surgery for morbid obesity is a major life-enhancing procedure for many obese patients. Many of these patients with morbid obesity experience significant psychiatric comorbidity, which requires comanagement along with the surgical care. The psychosomatic medicine team managed a case of complicated gastrointestinal bypass surgery in a bipolar disorder patient who had a prolonged period of nothing-by-mouth (NPO) status postoperatively. This represented a case of off-label psychopharmacological improvisation to manage the patient's psychiatric symptoms while in a long period of NPO status.

> The patient was a 25-year-old white female with morbid obesity and bipolar II disorder. Because of failure to control her weight and co-occurring sleep apnea syndrome and osteoarthritis, she was scheduled for gastric bypass surgery. Preoperatively, she had been stabilized on a regimen of bupropion 200 mg daily, paroxetine 40 mg daily, divalproex sodium 750 mg daily, topiramate 100 mg daily, and zolpidem 10 mg daily. Her last mood episode had been an episode of depression 2 years earlier. Her surgery initially appeared to go well, but in the early postoperative period she developed a failed anastomosis with leakage of gastric contents. Because of these complications, she was to

require 1 month of NPO status and total parenteral nutritional support. The psychosomatic medicine service was called to discuss psychotropic medication options in light of the NPO limitation.

On examination, she was in neither a depressed nor a hypomanic/manic episode but was anxious about her postoperative course and concerned that she would relapse into another mood episode if she could not receive ongoing psychopharmacological intervention. She was initially given lorazepam 1–2 mg intravenously every 4 hours as needed for anxiety, insomnia, or agitation. On this regimen, she became dysphoric and tearful. At this point, it was felt that she needed specific mood-stabilizer treatment. Because of her NPO status, she was started on intravenous valproate 250 mg three times a day. Within 3 days, she had much less affective lability and no further tearfulness. After consultation with the surgical team, olanzapine 2.5 mg orally disintegrating tablets twice daily were added.

Five days later, her serum valproate level was 34 μg/dL and her liver-associated enzymes were normal. She continued to be free of depressive and hypomanic/manic symptoms, had a normal sleep pattern, and was much less anxious than she had been. She was discharged on orally disintegrating olanzapine 2.5 mg twice a day and valproate 250 mg intravenously three times a day, with a recommendation to follow up with outpatient psychiatry and to increase the valproate dosage to 500 mg intravenously twice a day with a subsequent serum valproate level taken.

◆ **Diagnosis: Axis I—Bipolar II Disorder, 296.89; Delirium, 293.0**

This case represented a common comorbidity of mood disorder and morbid obesity. As with most major surgery, a brief period of interruption of oral psychotropic medications is expected in the immediate postoperative period. A dilemma may result, however, when surgical complications result in a prolonged period of NPO status, because the majority of psychotropic medications routinely used for bipolar disorder are only available in oral formulations. In this woman's case, she had been quite stable for 2 years on a somewhat complex psychopharmacological regimen. Postoperatively, a major concern for her (justifiably) was that interruption of her psychopharmacological regimen could provoke a depressive or hypomanic/manic relapse. Intravenous valproate, which is approved by the U.S. Food and Drug Administration for neurological indications such as seizure disorder, represented a creative alternative pathway to mood stabilization. Because she had tolerated oral valproate well preoperatively, it was reasonable to use intravenous valproate while she was NPO. To supplement the effects of valproate, orally disintegrating olanzapine was added. This was likely partially absorbed across the buccal mucosa for an additional effect, whereas the conventional dosage form of olanzapine would have required entirely intestinal absorption. Other options in such a dilemma include the use of intramuscular medications, such as immediate-release ziprasidone and olanzapine or depot risperidone, but the intravenous approach with valproate allowed the patient to avoid the pain and discomfort of intramuscular injections.

Recurrent Hepatic Encephalopathy: Intermittent/Chronic Delirium

The patient was a 57-year-old white man. He had a history of bipolar disorder, with onset in his 20s, which was stable on a maintenance dosage of lithium carbonate, 450 mg twice a day, with a therapeutic lithium serum level of 0.7 mEq/L. He had had no decompensation of his mood disorder in over 30 years. He also had a history of alcohol and drug abuse/dependence but no recent use of substances. Approximately 15 years earlier, he had undergone a course of interferon treatment for hepatitis C virus that was likely related to intravenous drug use. He eventually suffered progression of his liver disease to where he was on the borderline of being a liver transplantation candidate.

In a period of 4 months he had four admissions for hepatic encephalopathy. One of these episodes was precipitated by gallstone pancreatitis, whereas others were associated with systemic infections and/or periodic increases in his serum ammonia levels. During his acute presentations, which were somewhat stereotyped on each admission, he would be psychotic (hallucinating imaginary figures in his room) and agitated, with an inverted sleep-wake pattern (awake and agitated in the evenings and sleeping during the day) and profound cognitive impairment. His Mini-Mental State Examination (MMSE; Folstein et al. 1975) scores were less than 10. Fortunately, his renal function remained normal, so lithium carbonate was continued.

Aggressive management of his increased serum ammonia levels with lactulose and the addition of olanzapine, 20 mg at bedtime, to his maintenance lithium carbonate were associated with clearing of his delirium episodes within several days. With this treatment, his cognitive status improved to an MMSE score of 27 with full level of consciousness and no further psychotic symptoms. Because of the pattern of frequent recurrence of his delirium episodes, he was maintained on olanzapine and lithium with close outpatient follow-up.

In outpatient care, he was generally stable, without recurrence of severe cognitive or psychotic symptoms. However, his cognitive status showed mild fluctuations, which typically responded to brief increases in his lactulose dosages. Several months later, he developed glucose intolerance and was switched from olanzapine to aripiprazole 10 mg daily, which he tolerated well without any recurrence of mood or psychotic symptoms.

◆ **Diagnosis: Axis I—Bipolar Disorder Not Otherwise Specified, 296.80; Alcohol Dependence, 303.90; Opioid Dependence, 304.00; Delirium Due to Liver Disease, 293.0**

This case represents several interesting clinical phenomena. First, the patient had a history of bipolar disorder. On some of the admissions for delirium, despite the presentation in the context of liver disease, other physicians wondered if he was having repeated manic episodes (despite continued therapeutic doses of lithium). Manic episodes could be quickly eliminated from consideration by the absence of elated mood, no lack of need for sleep (although the sleep pattern was inverted from normal), and, as much as could be determined, no classic manic symptoms of pressured speech, goal-directed behavior, and sexual and social improprieties. Despite these differences, it was at times difficult to have colleagues appreciate the recurrent nature of the delirium, because they were prone to interpret any change in his mental status as representing destabilization of his bipolar disorder.

A second issue was trying to make the case for using the recurrent delirium episodes as a marker for hepatic failure and to thus potentially enhance this patient's liver transplant candidacy. This argument was not successful because it was not persuasive to the other members of the transplant service that a new liver would definitively preclude the recurrent delirium episodes. In addition, fortunately, the patient's renal function remained good, with normal creatinine level and electrolytes. Had he progressed to hepatorenal syndrome, the continued use of lithium would have been problematic.

Finally, because of the patient's recurrent pattern of delirium and his impaired cognitive status, even when recovered from the circadian disturbances, motor agitation, and psychotic symptoms at the height of his delirium episodes, he was maintained on an antipsychotic chronically. Delirium is usually thought of as a subacute- to acute- onset condition of limited duration. The construct of *chronic* or *intermittent* delirium, especially in patients with a continued state of metabolic compromise such as liver failure, facilitates the physician's thinking in continuing patients on antidelirium medications (e.g., antipsychotic agents) until there is a major change in the underlying condition, such as hepatic transplantation.

Somatic Gastrointestinal Delusion

A 50-year-old man with significant abdominal obesity was referred for psychosomatic medicine consultation due to psychotic symptoms. On examination, he related a spectacular delusional attribution of his significant obesity. His expanding girth, he explained, was due to "infestation." He believed that his abdomen had been invaded (through his umbilicus) by a pair of male and female "lobsters." The "lobsters" had then made their way from the umbilicus to the stomach, where ("like a tapeworm") they proceeded to "eat the food that I have eaten." Both "lobsters" gradually grew and eventually reproduced "baby lobsters" that perpetuated the cycle. The more the "lobsters" grew and reproduced, of course, the more he had to eat to sustain them, which led to more and more increased abdominal girth.

Curiously, he appeared not to have had a confirmed diagnosis of a psychotic disorder prior to the onset of the elaborate delusion (which, due the "marine life" theme, was dubbed a "psychquatic disorder" by a psychiatry resident working on his case). He had sought out care with several gastroenterologists with the specific request that they perform endoscopic examinations so as to remove the "lobsters." He was unwilling to entertain the possibility that his explanation might be inaccurate, despite the obvious failure to image the "lobsters" on radiographic studies. Several attempts to gently confront the delusional beliefs were not productive. He was offered antipsychotic medication, which he refused.

◆ **Diagnosis: Axis I—Psychotic Disorder Not Otherwise Specified, 298.9**

This case presents a remarkable delusional system that appeared to be generated as an "explanation" for the gradual increasing abdominal girth the patient was experiencing. The self-perpetuating nature of the delusional belief system (the "lobsters" were "eating" his ingested food and reproducing, thus "logically" requiring more food intake to sustain them) both reinforced the veracity of the original delusion and led to a ready explanation of the gradual increase in obesity over time. Although this patient resisted medication, one would prefer to attempt a trial of antipsychotic medication to treat the delusions. In such a case, the metabolic consequences of this delusion-affected obesity constrains treatment choices, because the obesity risk with olanzapine (and to a lesser degree, other atypical antipsychotic agents) renders these medications themselves problematic in obese, psychotic patients.

Hepatitis C Virus, Interferon, Transplantation, and Depression

The relationship between hepatitis C and depression is twofold: There is a higher incidence of depression in patients with hepatitis C (likely associated with the increased comorbidity of drug and alcohol abuse/dependence in many of these patients), and interferon/ribavirin treatment to treat hepatitis C is itself associated with mood disorders and other psychiatric phenomena (Crone and Gabriel 2003; Dieperink et al. 2000). This is an example in which the psychiatric comorbidity of a systemic illness and its specific therapy are "additive." Management of depression in hepatitis C patients is of twofold importance: 1) to enhance functioning of these patients with preexisting depression and 2) to treat interferon-associated mood disorders to enable successful navigation of a complex course of interferon to improve disease-free survival.

Case 1

The patient was a 35-year-old white man with a history of intravenous drug use who developed hepatitis C. When he was diagnosed with hepatitis C and the subsequent physical limitations became clear to him, he developed an episode of depression. He was treated with citalopram 20 mg orally every morning, with a good initial response. However, his hepatitis progressed to where he needed to go on interferon/ribavirin antiviral therapy. Three months into the therapy, his mood symptoms returned despite continued citalopram. His citalopram was then increased to 40 mg every morning. Within 1 month he was improved. He was maintained on citalopram for the 1-year duration of interferon/ribavirin treatment and then, because his mood was stable, slowly weaned and maintained under observation.

◆ **Diagnosis: Axis I—Polysubstance Dependence, 304.80; Depressive Disorder Not Otherwise Specified, 311**

Case 2

The patient was a 50-year-old Hispanic man with complaints of depressed mood, tearfulness, forgetfulness, poor concentration, variable sleep, appetite disturbance, and obsessionality for 1 month since beginning treatment with interferon/ribavirin for hepatitis C infection. He had no suicidality, homicidality, or psychosis. He was noted by his hepatologist to have a high score on a depression screening instrument at his hepatology appointment and was referred for outpatient psychosomatic medicine treatment. He had a history of alcohol dependence, including convictions for driving under the influence of alcohol, and past intravenous drug abuse, for which he had completed a recovery program with sustained abstinence. He had no other formal psychiatric history and had not previously received psychotropic medications.

His hepatitis C had been diagnosed 1 year previously, and its progression led to the need for interferon/ribavirin treatment. His systemic medical history was otherwise unremarkable. Despite his illness, he continued to work full-time and had a stable social support system in place.

On examination, he was mildly obese, with non-tearful and non-labile affect. His mental status examination revealed an MMSE score of 27. He was concerned about his hepatic status and somewhat embarrassed to discuss his mood symptoms, because he thought to be "depressed" in this context reflected "personal weakness." In a sense, he appeared more concerned over his mood symptoms than his liver disease. He was diagnosed with mood disorder, depressed type, secondary to interferon. He was treated with venlafaxine extended release, 75 mg every morning, and was seen in follow-up 1 month later.

On follow-up, he reported feeling much better. He had improved sleep and appetite and felt "sharper" cognitively, without any further disturbances in concentration or memory. He was tolerating venlafaxine well, with some mild dry mouth but good sexual function and no gastrointestinal symptoms. Repeat cognitive examination revealed that he now had intact short-term memory.

Unfortunately, he did not respond to interferon/ribavirin and had an increasing viral load. When seen for a second follow-up 1 month thereafter, he reported that he was initially distressed about the bad news regarding his treatment nonresponse, but he quickly reconstituted with help of his support network. After he mobilized his support network and came off of interferon and ribavirin, his mood symptoms remained improved. His mental status examination was unchanged. Because he was no longer receiving interferon and ribavirin, he wished to come off of venlafaxine. Venlafaxine was tapered and discontinued; he did not experience a recurrence of mood symptoms.

◆ **Diagnosis: Axis I—Mood Disorder Due to Interferon, 293.83; Opioid Abuse in Remission, 305.50; Alcohol Dependence in Remission, 303.90**

Case 3

The patient was a 50-year-old white man with a history of hepatitis C virus following intravenous drug abuse with concurrent alcohol dependence. He had had a liver transplant 2 years previously for progression of liver disease to cirrhosis. He had some difficulty dealing with his posttransplant adjustment and had developed depression with positive neurovegetative signs, for which he had not received psychiatric treatment.

Unfortunately, he had developed recurrent hepatitis C in the transplanted liver and was referred for a second course of interferon/ribavirin treatment. His hepatologist referred him for psychiatric treatment prior to beginning treatment, out of concern that the psychiatric side effects of interferon and ribavirin might exacerbate the patient's mood symptoms. He was not suicidal and had never had psychotic symptoms. He continued to attend Alcoholics Anonymous meetings to maintain his recovery. His only current medication was tacrolimus. On examination, he appeared mildly dysphoric, nontearful, and nonlabile. He had normal cognitive status with an MMSE score of 30. Because of his current depressive symptoms and the impending course of interferon and ribavirin, he was started on venlafaxine extended release, 75 mg daily.

When seen in follow-up 2 months later, the patient was tolerating his venlafaxine well. His mood was better, and his sleep and appetite were now normal. He remained without suicidal ideation or psychotic symptoms. He noted mild dry mouth but no neurological or sexual side effects from venlafaxine. Most importantly, he was able to tolerate the trial of interferon and ribavirin well and expected to be able to complete the requisite months of antiviral therapy. Examination revealed less dysphoric, nontearful, nonlabile affect. He was instructed to complete a 12-month course of venlafaxine, corresponding to the anticipated course of interferon and ribavirin.

◆ **Diagnosis: Axis I—Mood Disorder Due to Interferon, 293.83; Opioid Abuse in Remission, 305.50; Alcohol Dependence in Remission, 303.90**

Mood symptoms, predominantly depression, are commonly reported in the context of interferon and ribavirin treatment for hepatitis C virus infection (Crone and Gabriel 2003; Dieperink et al. 2000). In addition, with the majority of hepatitis C infections occurring in intravenous drug abusers, there is a likelihood of depression associated with substance abuse in these patients as well. These mechanisms obviously take into full account the psychodynamic issue of depression associated with the sense of physical and existential threat represented by a serious and life-threatening illness. Even in a successful case of interferon/ribavirin-responsive hepatitis C, there is requisite compliance for 1 year (often longer) with medications that have significant systemic side effects. Untreated mood disorder symptoms in this context can lead directly to noncompliance, further compromising the response to antiviral treatment, in an unfortunate and progressive spiral. Thus, depression in hepatitis C is an excellent model for the utility of the psychosomatic medicine approach.

Case 1 above illustrates that intervention with antidepressant medication can result in a clinical response for hepatitis C–associated depression. When treating hepatitis patients, one should remain aware of the status of the illness and its treatment. When compensated depressive patients with hepatitis C then go on to interferon/ribavirin therapy, particular attention is warranted. Antidepressants may be maintained throughout the course of interferon/ribavirin to guard against rebound mood symptoms.

The second patient, despite his substance abuse history, did not have a mood disorder diagnosis until 1 month after starting interferon/ribavirin; indeed, he handled the news of needing to go on interferon/ribavirin without a contemporary change in mood. Only when he was 1 month into treatment did he develop mood symptoms.

Astute monitoring of his mood state by his hepatologist led to prompt referral and treatment. He had a robust clinical response within several weeks of starting venlafaxine, with reversal of his mood symptoms. Unfortunately, his nonresponse to interferon and ribavirin led to these medications being discontinued. When the interferon and ribavirin were discontinued, he was then able to discontinue venlafaxine without recurrence of depression symptoms, supporting the inference that the mood symptoms were medication related.

The third patient presented with depression 2 years after his liver transplant operation and, unfortunately, had had a recurrence of hepatitis C that necessitated a course of interferon/ribavirin to treat the transplanted liver. Similarly to the patient in Case 1, this patient's depression before starting interferon/ribavirin led his hepatologist to request that his depression be fully treated before starting antiviral treatment. In this man's case, compliance both with the immunosuppressive medication to preserve the liver transplant and antiviral treatment to suppress the hepatitis C made treatment of depression and maximal medication and clinical care compliance imperative. As with the first case, he had a good clinical response to venlafaxine, with improved mood, and he was then able to proceed with interferon/ribavirin in an improved condition.

Care of hepatitis C patients in the various stages of illness, from diagnosis through interferon/ribavirin treatment, and sometimes through the process of liver transplantation, serves as fertile ground for psychosomatic medicine physicians to closely collaborate with physician colleagues in the integrative and multidisciplinary care of these unfortunate patients.

Psychosis About Food With Wasting

The patient was a 55-year-old white man with schizophrenia, paranoid type. He had been hospitalized at a mental health facility for several weeks but began to refuse feedings and was transferred to a university medical center. He received intravenous fluids and was stabilized. A psychosomatic medicine consultation was called for management of his psychosis. On examination, he shared a typical story of paranoid schizophrenia with chronic auditory hallucinations and delusional beliefs. However, his psychosis had taken a remarkable turn that explained his new-onset refusal of food.

The reason he had begun to refuse food at the psychiatric facility was, he said, because their food was contaminated. Not with poisons or food-borne illnesses-causing microbes, but with "little steel airplanes, about a half inch long. Listen, you can hear them flying around." Whereupon, he held his spoon in front of his ear and told the examiner how he "heard" the "airplanes." "I can't eat food with airplanes in it—I would break my teeth!"

This remarkable delusion presented a clinical dilemma. Until he was taking oral feeds, he was not medically stable for transfer to an inpatient psychiatric facility. Until he was less psychotic, he was not going to eat adequately. He was also unwilling to take antipsychotic medications in the medical center. A temporary solution was tube feedings; he was not delusional about the tube feedings containing "airplanes." Later, after many negotiations and reassurances of its safety, he tolerated a "pureed" diet, because his perception was that the mechanical processing of the pureed diet made it safe. Eventually, he was stabilized on the pureed diet to where he was medically stable for return to the mental health facility.

◆ **Diagnosis: Axis I—Schizophrenia, Paranoid Type, 295.30**

This man's paranoid delusions about his food led to a refusal to take adequate nutrition. Because he would not maintain an adequate diet, he needed inpatient medical attention. His "airplanes" delusion was quite persistent and, to him, frightening. His refusal to take psychotropic medications accentuated his condition. We were left with little to offer him but an empathic stance and a willingness to explore his concerns and to negotiate a manner of food preparation that he would regard as safe to eat.

Pancreatic Encephalopathy

The patient was a 64-year-old white man with a negative psychiatric history. He had experienced 2 days of escalating abdominal pain and confusion. When he was initially seen at a community hospital, his amylase and lipase were elevated to 4,156 U/L and 8,195 U/L, respectively, and he was transferred to an academic medical center for management of pancreatitis. Upon admission, he had altered mental status (consisting of agitation, paranoid ideation, hallucinating his wife's voice, confusion, and disorientation) and elevated amylase and lipase of 774 U/L and 187 U/L, respectively. Computed tomography scans confirmed pancreatitis. He was diagnosed with delirium. The psychosomatic medicine team recommended the use of antipsychotic medications, but the intensive care service admitting him refused to order antipsychotics, not wanting to "cloud his mental status further." Although it was frustrating to have medication recommendations not followed regarding psychotropic medications, this did afford the opportunity to see the "natural history" of delirium due to pancreatic encephalopathy unfold.

The patient's amylase and lipase normalized by hospital day 4, but his mental status changes persisted for 11 more days. He was unable to score any points on the MMSE until day 12, when he scored a 9; on that day, he also had perseverative speech and continued confusion; for example, he claimed that his illness was due to his "testtestosterone [sic] gland." Finally, on hospital day 15, he was no longer agitated nor was he as confused. He was then able to recall a recent visit from his wife and was able to reconstruct some of the memories of his delirium episode; for instance, he recalled being frightened by having artwork on the hospital room wall "speak" to him. He continued steady improvement in his mental status, and his MMSE score finally returned to the unimpaired range by hospital day 19.

♦ **Diagnosis: Axis I—Delirium, 293.0**

Pancreatic encephalopathy is an infrequently reported syndrome of acute and severe delirium in the context of acute pancreatitis (Estrada et al. 1979). Several cases with extremely poor outcomes (including fatalities) have been reported. The presumed mechanism remains in question; it has been suggested that fat emboli from the acute pancreatic injury may be responsible for central nervous system vascular events. Other metabolic factors such as central nervous system toxicity from liberated pancreatic enzymes, increased cerebrospinal fluid lipase, hypoxia from pulmonary fat emboli, and aberrant urea cycle metabolism may all be in play. Psychosomatic medicine physicians should consider the diagnosis of pancreatic encephalopathy when encountering severe acute delirium in the setting of acute pancreatitis.

Compulsive Foreign Body Ingestion

It is likely that among the most troubling patients for the gastroenterologist and surgeon is the patient with compulsive foreign body ingestion. We have treated several such patients, all of whom were prisoners.

Case 1

The first of these patients was a 35-year-old man. He was in the habit of impulsively ingesting foreign objects when upset or angry. He denied specific suicidal intent, although he described a need to "punish" himself with these ingestions. He was treated within the prison system for borderline personality disorder; his treatment included divalproex and psychotherapy. Another motivation for this behavior was that ingestion of these foreign objects would get him temporarily out of prison and to the medical center, a far more pleasant social environment.

He was admitted after yet another such ingestion. While angry at prison officials for a nonspecific administrative slight, he had grabbed a dozen ballpoint pens and, before custody officers could restrain him, swallowed them. He was emergently admitted to the surgery service. Abdominal X-ray revealed the pens in his stomach, all pointing toward the gastric antrum. They were removed endoscopically without complications.

After the procedure, the patient was interviewed by the psychosomatic medicine service. He was not psychotic, and his mood was only mildly irritable. He did not appear to have a significant mood disorder. He told us readily that when "stressed" he felt a need to "punish" himself by eating a foreign object. He denied specifically wanting to kill himself but did say he wanted to "induce pain" in himself. At some other times, he could offer no explanation for this ingestion of foreign objects, saying that he just "had" to do it. The nature of these ingestions in response to nonspecific stressors is consistent with borderline personality disorder. After his recovery, he was transferred back to the prison system.

◆ **Diagnosis: Axis I—Borderline Personality Disorder, 301.83**

Case 2

The second case was a 44-year-old African American man. He was admitted for gastrointestinal surgery after having swallowed several razor blades several days earlier. He was serving a life sentence for multiple felony convictions and had been transferred several times within the prison system. He described a history of compulsive foreign body ingestion beginning at age 8, when he began "licking the rust off of nails." This habit progressed to where he would frequently swallow metal objects, typically during a period of stress or abandonment.

He had had a very impoverished and abusive childhood. His drug-abusing mother and stepfather would repeatedly beat and humiliate him. After his mother lost custody of him due to her drug use, he was raised primarily by his grandmother and great-aunt. He had had several psychiatric hospitalizations as a youth for acting-out behavior and was variously diagnosed with attention-deficit/hyperactivity disorder, psychotic disorder, and borderline personality disorder. He had intermittent hallucinations, consisting of intrusive voices that "said" critical comments about his behavior and "commanded" him to consume metal objects as punishment.

He had many periods of feeling depressed, lonely, and painfully abandoned; during such mood states he would find paradoxical relief in the pain caused by swallowing a sharp object, as though the physical pain from the sharp object was more tolerable than the psychic pain he would otherwise experience. As an adult, due to his criminal behavior, he had been in prison for 20 years with no hope of release. When finally able, in the prison system, to obtain regular psychiatric care, he was treated with bupropion, oxcarbazepine, divalproex, and haloperidol. These medications offered some symptomatic relief from his mood and psychotic symptoms, but when under distress, he would continue to swallow foreign objects.

By age 44, he had endured several gastrointestinal surgeries to retrieve these swallowed objects. Upon yet another prison transfer, he lost his access to his regular treating psychiatrist. Under the distress of this abandonment, he then swallowed the razor blades that generated the admission. On examination, he had dysphoric, labile affect but was not currently suicidal or homicidal, nor did he endorse current psychotic symptoms. He was kept on a suicide watch; postoperatively, he was restarted on his regular medications and was transferred back to the prison.

♦ **Diagnosis: Axis I—Psychotic Disorder Not Otherwise Specified, 298.9; Axis II—Borderline Personality Disorder, 301.83**

Such patients, especially when they have had several admissions for repeated foreign body ingestion, will often cause enormous negative countertransference feelings in treating physicians, nurses, and other staff members. These patients are often best understood as primitive borderline personality disorder with a compulsion for self-damaging acting out, especially when anxious or angry (Groves 1975, 1978). Assisting the medical staff in appropriate treatment of the patient while fully acknowledging these strong feeling states and assisting with a more empathic approach to these patients is very important.

In encounters with the patient, safety must first be assured. If these patients are already in legal custody, the custody officers must be vigilant for additional impulsive ingestions, to the point of not providing the patient with materials that would ordinarily be considered routine and even "humane" (e.g., silverware, writing tools, paper). If such patients are not in legal custody, constant supervision (even in the bathroom) within "arm's length" distance is essential. Medications to decrease impulsive behavior (e.g., antipsychotics, antidepressants, and mood stabilizers) can be considered.

Clozapine- and Benztropine-Associated Ileus

The patient was a 50-year-old single man with a 30-year history of paranoid schizophrenia characterized by hallucinations, delusions, disorganization, negative symptoms, and marginal social function. He had been treated with a large number of psychotropic medications in various combinations over the years, and at the time of admission was taking clozapine 600 mg daily, benztropine 4 mg daily, and fluoxetine 20 mg daily. He had had no recent psychiatric hospitalizations and had been on stable dosages of his medications for more than a year.

He then experienced a gradual onset and progressive series of gastrointestinal symptoms. He had a decreased appetite associated with constipation and increasing abdominal pain. Gradually, he developed abdominal distention and vomiting. He was admitted emergently to the university medical center. Evaluation revealed a distended abdomen with minimal bowel sounds, and abdominal imaging revealed dilated loop of bowel with air fluid levels, diagnostic of intestinal obstruction.

Conservative management with nasogastric tube placement for decompression, pain relief, and intravenous hydration were unsuccessful. He underwent a successful partial resection of a portion of small bowel. Postoperatively, he regained bowel function over several days and was able to be restarted on psychotropic medication. Clozapine was held and quetiapine 600 mg daily was started instead, benztropine was discontinued, and fluoxetine was continued. Thereafter, he was transferred to an inpatient psychiatry unit for continued care.

♦ **Diagnosis: Axis I—Schizophrenia, Paranoid Type, 295.30; Adverse Effects of Medication Not Otherwise Specified, 995.2**

Clozapine is the antipsychotic often reserved for the most problematic cases of unremitting psychotic illness. Although the rare side effect of agranulocytosis is well known, appropriately screened for, and monitored cautiously by psychiatrists, the less acutely dangerous receptor side effects of clozapine may also be clinically significant.

In this patient's case, the formulation of the genesis of his small bowel obstruction relates to medication-induced dysmotility. First, clozapine is significantly anticholinergic, as much so as many tricyclic antidepressants and low-potency first-generation antipsychotic medications. This effect alone may adequately account for this man's presentation; indeed, postoperatively, we felt it unsafe to rechallenge him with clozapine. Second, clozapine has significant α-adrenergic effects, so when the patient began to experience dehydration due to compromised gastrointestinal function leading to decreased intravascular volume, he may consequently have had additional problems with delirium.

Third, he was concurrently receiving benztropine, which is itself significantly anticholinergic, thus creating an additive anticholinergic effect. Finally, there was the drug–drug interaction between fluoxetine and clozapine. Due to fluoxetine's inhibition of the cytochrome P450 2D6 isoenzyme, co-administered fluoxetine can increase the serum levels of clozapine by 50%. Quetiapine does not feature this drug–drug interaction with fluoxetine and has minimal anticholinergic effects, so it was used postoperatively instead of clozapine (Sandson et al. 2005). Therefore, the effective anticholinergic effect of clozapine in the patient was potentiated by several additive factors.

Psychosomatic medicine psychiatrists need to be very cautious in the use of clozapine in medically ill patients. Clozapine should be considered among the other highly anticholinergic medications routinely limited in medically ill and delirium-prone patients (e.g., diphenhydramine, tricyclic antidepressants, and low-potency first-generation antipsychotics); the discontinuation of anticholinergic medications is especially crucial in cases of reduced gastrointestinal motility, because cholinergic blockade is an important cause of bowel dysmotility. Caution regarding the combining of anticholinergic psychotropic medications is also important. Finally, attention to drug–drug interactions among psychotropic medications that have the undesirable net effect of increasing anticholinergic toxicity needs to be integrated into the psychosomatic intervention as well.

References

Black DW, Goldstein RB, Mason EE: Prevalence of mental disorder in 88 morbidly obese bariatric clinic patients. Am J Psychiatry 149:227–234, 1992

Clark MM, Balkier BM, Slattern CD, et al: Psychosocial factors and 2-year outcome following bariatric surgery for weight loss. Obes Surg 13:739–745, 2003

Clark MM, Hanna BK, Mai JL, et al: Sexual abuse survivors and psychiatric hospitalization after bariatric surgery. Obes Surg 17:465–469, 2007

Crone C, Gabriel GM: Comprehensive review of hepatitis C for psychiatrists: risks, screening, diagnosis, treatment, and interferon-based therapy complications. J Psychiatr Pract 9:93–110, 2003

Dieperink E, Willenbring M, Ho SB: Neuropsychiatric symptoms associated with hepatitis C and interferon alpha: a review. Am J Psychiatry 157:867–876, 2000

Estrada RV, Moreno J, Martinez E, et al: Pancreatic encephalopathy. Acta Neurol Scand 59:135–139, 1979

Folstein MF, Folstein SE, McHugh PR: "Mini-Mental State": a practical method for grading the cognitive state of patients for the clinician. J Psychiatr Res 12:189–198, 1975

Griffith JL, Gaby L: Brief psychotherapy at the bedside: countering demoralization from medical illness. Psychosomatics 46:109–116, 2005

Grothe KB, Dubbert, PM, O'Jile JR: Psychological assessment and management of the weight loss surgery patient. Am J Med Sci 331:201–206, 2006

Groves JE: Management of the borderline patient on a medical or surgical ward: the psychiatric consultant's role. Int J Psychiatry Med 6:337–348, 1975

Groves JE: Taking care of the hateful patient. N Engl J Med 298:883–887, 1978

Herpertz S, Kiel Mann R, Wolf AM, et al: Do psychosocial variables predict weight loss or mental health after obesity surgery? A systematic review. Obes Res 12:1554–1569, 2004

Hsu LKG, Menotti PN, Dwyer J, et al: No surgical factors that influence the outcome of bariatric surgery: a review. Psychosis Med 60:338–346, 1998

Powers PS, Perez A, Boyd F, et al: Eating pathology before and after bariatric surgery: a prospective study. Int J Eat Disord 25:293–300, 1999

Sandson NB, Armstrong SC, Cozza KL: An overview of psychotropic drug–drug interactions. Psychosomatics 46:464–494, 2005

Sarwer DB, Cohn MI, Gobbons LM, et al: Psychiatric diagnosis and psychiatric treatment among bariatric surgery candidates. Obes Surg 14:1148–1156, 2004

Sarwer DB, Warden TA, Fabricator AN: Psychosocial and behavioral aspects of bariatric surgery. Obes Res 13:639–648, 2005

Segal A, Kinoshita-Kussunoki D, Aparecida Larino M: Post-surgical refusal to eat: anorexia nervosa, bulimia nervosa or a new eating disorder? A case series. Obes Surg 14:353–357, 2004

Sogg S, Mor DL: The Boston Interview for Gastric Bypass: determining the psychological suitability of surgical candidates. Obes Surg 14:370–380, 2004

6

RENAL DISEASE

The connection between renal disease and psychosomatic medicine is important for many reasons. Renal disease requiring dialysis support is frequently accompanied by depression and fatigue. Whether this is primarily due to associated anemia or a sense of helplessness and dependency on dialysis machines for life-sustaining treatment is often unclear, and certainly many patients appear to have both of these factors in play. In addition, mentally ill patients, by dint of their psychiatric symptoms, may be less able to cope with the behavioral expectations of renal dialysis. Patients treated with lithium carbonate are at risk for either acute (often resulting from overdose) or chronic renal toxicity after lithium therapy; such patients must thereafter be managed with other medications. Finally, kidney transplant surgery requires behavioral stability and compliance; psychosomatic medicine psychiatrists are often intimately involved in renal transplant teams managing these patients.

"God Has Healed My Kidneys"

We recently managed a bipolar disorder patient with dialysis dependence for whom acceptance of dialysis itself was compromised by the nature of her delusional belief system. Solving this case required the creative application of several clinical approaches.

> A 67-year-old white woman with long-standing bipolar disorder and end-stage renal disease was admitted to an inpatient psychiatric facility during an acute manic episode with psychotic features. She was prescribed aripiprazole 30 mg, olanzapine 5 mg, and valproic acid 1,000 mg, all to be given at bedtime. She also received lorazepam

0.5 mg every 8 hours as needed for agitation. While in the psychiatric facility, staff members were unable to persuade the patient to attend her thrice-weekly hemodialysis sessions. After 2 weeks of dialysis refusal, the patient became mildly confused and ataxic and was transferred to the emergency department of a university medical center for emergent hemodialysis.

The psychosomatic medicine service was called to see the patient in the emergency department to assess her decisional capacity to refuse hemodialysis and to help manage her bipolar disorder. On initial evaluation, the patient reported that she did not want to continue hemodialysis because the "bumps" on her arm were "not very feminine." She also denied that renal failure was a problem for her anymore, because "God has healed my kidneys."

The patient was noted to have pressured speech and an irritable mood; her Mini-Mental State Examination (MMSE; Folstein et al. 1975) score was 24. Her initial serum blood urea nitrogen was 120 mg/dL, her creatinine level was 5.7 mg/dL, and her potassium was 4.6 mEq/L. The psychiatrist recommended use of a surrogate decision maker because the delusional denial of her renal failure impaired the patient's capacity to appreciate the risks and benefits of refusing hemodialysis. Although a close friend acting as surrogate consented for dialysis, the mere declaration of incapacity for consent did not confer behavioral control in itself. The patient frequently became agitated when taken to the hospital dialysis suite and returned undialyzed to her room because dialysis personnel were not willing to physically restrain her to perform the procedure.

Premedication of the patient before dialysis with lorazepam 0.5 mg and olanzapine 10 mg in orally dissolving form was then recommended and resulted in several successful hemodialysis sessions. Although the patient continued to be intrusive and irritable, her MMSE score rose to 29 after hemodialysis.

Prior to the onset of renal failure, the patient had been treated for many years with lithium carbonate as well as several other psychotropic medications. She lived in a board and care facility and, with this structure and supervision, she had been able to avoid repeated psychiatric hospitalizations and was largely behaviorally stable on her medication. However, in combination with a partial nephrectomy for renal cell carcinoma, the years of lithium carbonate had taken their renal toll, and she developed end-stage renal failure. This became quickly problematic in two ways. She could no longer be treated with lithium carbonate, which had effectively maintained her psychiatric status for many years, and she needed to cooperate behaviorally with the dialysis regimen required to treat the renal failure.

For 3 years prior to the current admission, hemodialysis clinic personnel reported tolerating frequent agitated and uncooperative behavior by the patient. She would disturb and frighten other dialysis patients and threaten to pull out intravenous lines and to leave the dialysis clinic. Although she often missed dialysis sessions, the patient did maintain enough consistency to avoid fluid overload and uremic encephalopathy. However, because of her behavior the patient was at risk of losing her "spot" in the clinic.

After medical stabilization, the patient was returned to the inpatient psychiatric unit. Premedication with an antipsychotic agent immediately before dialysis treatments helped her to avoid agitation. This regimen was continued after discharge with the expectation that further outpatient hemodialysis sessions would proceed without issue.

◆ **Diagnosis: Axis I—Bipolar I Disorder, Most Recent Episode Manic, Severe With Psychotic Features, 296.44; Delirium (Resolved), 293.0**

The challenges of dealing with chronic renal failure leading to dialysis dependency are profound for many patients; witness the high rates of depression seen in dialysis-dependent patients. The daily reminders of mortality, the thrice-weekly obligatory visits to the dialysis suite for several hours of life-maintaining treatment, and the sense of dependency on "the machine" and on the medical care system are obvious. Less dramatic but of similar importance are the loss of a sense of productivity because of the time spent either acutely ill or undergoing dialysis treatment and the often disabling fatigue from the anemia associated with renal failure.

All these psychological factors are present in many dialysis patients. However, when the patient also has a significant major psychiatric illness, there are additional complications and challenges that will promptly come to the attention of the psychosomatic medicine psychiatrist. This patient's bipolar disorder, previously reasonably well compensated on lithium and an antipsychotic, destabilized when renal failure required that lithium be discontinued. In addition, her emerging psychotic thinking about "divine intervention" for her kidneys and her agitation in the dialysis suite presented significant clinical management challenges.

Renal dialysis units must function efficiently and safely to provide chronic care to patients. Dialysis units cannot be expected to tolerate agitated, psychotic, and otherwise disruptive patients. Hence, getting chronically mentally ill patients placed in a dialysis model may be problematic. The treating nephrologist and dialysis unit staff need plausible reassurance that patients will not act out in dialysis suites. Patients with concurrent bipolar disorder, schizoaffective disorder, or schizophrenia and dialysis dependence may not be readily accepted by inpatient psychiatric facilities because of the need to transport and supervise patients for regular dialysis treatments. Therefore, when such patients are in the general hospital and simultaneously in need of psychiatric stabilization and ongoing dialysis treatment, initiating a psychiatric commitment process may not be possible.

Similarly, patients may refuse dialysis for psychotic reasons, as in this case. In such times, surrogate consent may be needed to continue with dialysis. The underlying major psychiatric illness must be managed with medications other than lithium carbonate. We have found that generous use of atypical antipsychotic agents (subject to the usual cautions to their use), particularly sedating agents such as olanzapine, dosed immediately before dialysis treatments, helps to safely sedate dialysis patients to tolerate the procedure. Chronically mentally ill patients with a need for dialysis may need to have their poor insight into their renal disease and frank denial of the need for dialysis taken into account in legal proceedings to determine their capacity for appropriate self-care decisions.

Syndrome of Inappropriate Secretion of Antidiuretic Hormone From Serotonergic Psychotropic Medications

We have treated patients with syndrome of inappropriate secretion of antidiuretic hormone (SIADH) and hyponatremia associated with the use of serotonergic antidepressants, one with citalopram, another with venlafaxine, and a third with olanzapine.

Case 1

The first patient was a 70-year-old white male with mild vascular dementia and depression. He had no other psychiatric history. He had medical history significant for coronary artery disease with myocardial infarction, prostatic hypertrophy with transurethral resection of the prostate, hypertension, hyperlipidemia, hypothyroidism, and oropharyngeal carcinoma. He was started on citalopram 10 mg daily by his primary care physician.

Shortly after initiation of citalopram, the patient's mental status worsened noticeably, with increased anxiety and mood symptoms. Serum sodium decreased to 126 mEq/L. The patient presented with mild delirium; serum and urine osmolalities of 275 mOsm/kg and 460 mOsm/kg, respectively, and urine sodium of 131 mEq/L confirmed SIADH. After citalopram was discontinued, his sodium quickly increased to 134 mEq/L, and his mental status improved. On psychosomatic medicine evaluation he demonstrated mild tangentiality and an MMSE score of 21 with mild deficits in time orientation, recall memory, and concentration. He was pleasant and cooperative with euthymic and mood congruent affect.

◆ **Diagnosis: Axis I—Delirium, 293.0; Vascular Dementia, With Depressed Mood, 290.43; Depressive Disorder Not Otherwise Specified, 311**

Case 2

The second patient was a 75-year-old female with non–small cell carcinoma of the lung who was prescribed venlafaxine extended release 37.5 mg daily for depression that developed 6 months after her cancer diagnosis; in this time period she had received chemotherapy and cranial irradiation. After 1 week of venlafaxine therapy, her serum sodium decreased from a baseline of 132 mEq/L to 122 mEq/L, and she presented to the clinic with cognitive impairment and lethargy.

On psychosomatic medicine interview, she revealed blunted affect, no evidence of psychosis, and an MMSE score of 20. Her venlafaxine was stopped, and the sodium increased to 130 mEq/L within 6 days. Her cognitive status cleared to baseline levels when the sodium level increased.

◆ **Diagnosis: Axis I—Delirium, 293.0; Major Depressive Disorder, Single Episode, Severe Without Psychotic Features, 296.23**

Case 3

The third patient was a 50-year-old white female with a history of schizophrenia and long-term cigarette smoking. She was admitted from a psychiatric facility for shortness of breath. Workup revealed a cavitated lung mass and three cortical lesions, likely representing lung cancer with metastatic disease. Serum sodium was 125 mEq/L with serum osmolality of 264 mOsm/kg and urine osmolality of 152 mOsm/kg.

On examination she exhibited prominent negative symptoms, thought concreteness, and poor understanding of her illness. Her olanzapine was maintained at 15 mg am, 20 mg hs, and she was kept on fluid restriction. In this case, it is unclear whether the olanzapine, lung cancer, or central nervous system metastases were individually or collectively responsible for her SIADH.

♦ **Diagnosis: Axis I—Schizophrenia, Paranoid Type, 295.30**

These cases illustrate SIADH, a clinically significant problem affecting the renal system that is sometimes the consequence of the use of serotonergic agents (Kirby and Ames 2001). Psychotropic medications are responsible for a large percentage of medication-associated SIADH; therefore, prompt determination of urine and serum osmolalities are imperative when encountering euvolemic hyponatremia in a patient receiving serotonergic psychotropic medications. Conversely, serum electrolytes could be determined before routine use of serotonergic agents; any onset of apparent acute mental status changes following the use of serotonergic medications should lead to consideration of SIADH and require determination of serum electrolytes and urine and serum osmolalities. Patients with other systemic risk factors for SIADH, such as prior episodes of SIADH, lung disease, central nervous system pathology, and malignancy may be at additive risk for SIADH when serotonergic psychotropic medications are used.

Renal Failure, Diabetes Insipidus, and Persistence of Lithium Toxicity

Lithium toxicity has numerous systemic effects. Psychosomatic medicine physicians will often encounter patients with lithium toxicity, either after intentional lithium overdose or with a more ambiguous presentation unrelated to suicide attempts. The renal complications of lithium toxicity may acutely lead to severe disturbances in electrolyte status that may significantly compromise patient outcomes.

The patient was a 55-year-old African American female who had a history of severe bipolar disorder. She was taking lithium carbonate

450 mg daily and divalprocx sodium 1,500 mg daily. She had had numerous psychiatric hospitalizations for mood decompensation episodes. She was a resident of a board and care facility. She presented to the emergency department with confusion and tremors.

On examination, she was oriented in three spheres but had impaired recall memory and concentration. She was not suicidal or homicidal. She had no psychotic symptoms. Her level of consciousness was variable, and she became somnolent by the end of the interview. Serum lithium level was 2.4 mEq/L, Na^+ was 143 mEq/L, and her creatinine was 2.3 mg/dL. Computed tomography of the head revealed mild diffuse cortical atrophy. She was admitted to the intensive care unit for management of lithium toxicity. She did not receive hemodialysis. Her valproate was continued (with close monitoring of liver associated enzymes, serum valproate level, and ammonia level) to treat her underlying bipolar disorder.

By the next day, her condition had worsened. She could not be aroused to verbal stimuli and had had copious urine output. Her Na^+ level had (in 24 hours) increased to 168 mEq/L and her creatinine and lithium levels were now 2.3 mg/dL and 2.2 mEq/L, respectively. Her intravenous fluids, initially normal saline, were changed to deliver more free water. Diuretics were started; eventually she was able to maintain a normal serum Na^+ level.

However, after her several days of hypernatremia, her cognitive status had worsened. Some of the original signs of delirium had improved, to where she had a full level of consciousness and normal sleep-wake cycle, but she was now nonverbal. She would readily smile in apparent recognition when the examiner entered her hospital room, and she did not appear dysphoric, agitated, or irritable. She made some nonlinguistic utterances and could not reliably nod or shake her head to answer "yes/no" queries.

This patient had a severe diabetes insipidus episode following her lithium toxicity episode. The profound loss of free water had led to a dilutional hypernatremia. Despite management with intravenous fluids, diuretics, and close monitoring of her electrolytes, she experienced several episodes of recurrence of hypernatremia. Correspondingly, her creatinine was slow to normalize, and her lithium was slow to clear as well. She still had a lithium level of 0.3 mEq/L on hospital day 8, 9 days after her last lithium dose.

Several days after her lithium level was no longer detectable and her creatinine improved, she developed new neuropsychiatric findings. Although exhibiting a normal level of consciousness, no motor agitation, and no apparent disturbance in her circadian rhythms, she was now largely nonverbal. She would readily respond when approached, and she nodded "yes" when asked if she recognized familiar interviewers, but she would otherwise speak in only brief, one-word utterances. She did not exhibit motor agitation and did not appear depressed or manic. A magnetic resonance imaging scan at this time revealed possible demyelination of the anterior corpus callosum. Electroencephalography revealed continued bilateral diffuse slowing without evidence of seizure activity. Other neurological causes of her persistently regressed state were ruled out.

◆ **Diagnosis: Axis I—Bipolar I Disorder, Most Recent Episode Unspecified, 296.7; Delirium, 293.0; Adverse Effects of Medication Not Otherwise Specified, 995.2**

This unfortunate case illustrates some of the significant potential systemic renal and neurological signs of lithium toxicity. On first presentation, the patient appeared to have relatively unremarkable lithium toxicity. Notably, there was no evidence of suicidal intent or intentionality of overdose; indeed, because she had had her medications dispensed daily at her board and care facility (the case history showed no suspicion of her having acquired lithium surreptitiously from another source), an overdose was very unlikely.

Once she was admitted, she promptly developed diabetes insipidus and profound hypernatremia, a likely renal consequence of the subacute to acute lithium toxicity state. This was managed by switching from normal saline to hypotonic saline and with the use of diuretics. Notably, because her creatinine remained elevated, her lithium level required several days to be totally eliminated from her system; it is likely that the continued lithium exposure may have potentiated the renal lithium toxicity.

Finally, and most concerning, was her apparently persistent regressed status after her lithium had been eliminated and her hypernatremia fully resolved. There are some case reports of persistent neuropsychiatric impairment for lithium toxicity itself that, unfortunately, persists for an indefinite period even after complete clearance of lithium from the body. This is in contrast to the more familiar acute symptoms of lithium toxicity, which in most cases are completely reversible after elimination of lithium.

Psychiatrists are reminded, by virtue of this case, of the acute dangers of lithium toxicity—the renal effects of the toxicity that paradoxically impair the ability of the renal system to detoxify the remaining lithium, and the persistent effects on the central nervous system of this very important, but frequently dangerous, psycho-pharmacological agent.

Renal Failure From Therapeutic Use of Lithium

Lithium salts are, of course, an epoch-making advance for treatment of manic states. However, they are fraught with systemic complications. The psychosomatic medicine psychiatrist is frequently confronted with the patient who requires aggressive psychopharmacological care for severe bipolar disorder but who also experiences medically complicated systemic side effects from lithium. This requires a several-pronged approach. Alternative psychopharmacology (which must itself be systemically tolerable) to lithium must be substituted, the systemic side effects of lithium may need management, and the cumulative effects of lithium toxicity may lead to irreversible complications. All of these aspects may be present simultaneously.

> The patient was a 50-year-old single white male. He had had the onset of bipolar I disorder at age 19. His mood episodes consisted of classic manic episodes with decreased need for sleep, grandiosity and inflated self-esteem, and psychotic symptoms (with delusions of grandiosity). Between the disabling manic episodes, he struggled to maintain good social function but had been able to complete bachelor's and master's degrees and had been able to remain employed in retail management. Over the years, he had had 12 psychiatric hospitalizations, had received a single course of electroconvulsive therapy, and had been treated with numerous psychopharmacological agents. His best clinical response had been to lithium, which he received from his 20s until his late 40s, when he had had to discontinue its use because of lithium-induced renal impairment. He had never taken a lithium overdose, nor had he had discrete episodes of acute lithium toxicity.
>
> He had no other psychiatric illness and no substance abuse. Despite his severe mood disorder, he was very compliant with medications and other psychiatric treatments. After he was forced to discontinue lithium, he was maintained on divalproex sodium 1,000 mg, zolpidem 10 mg, and trazodone 50 mg, all at bedtime; on this combination he was able to avoid psychiatric hospitalization for 6 years. Unfortunately, his renal failure progressed despite his having discontinued lithium, and he eventually became dialysis dependent.
>
> The patient pursued renal transplantation and relocated to California temporarily to stay with his sister, who also served as the kidney

donor. On clinical examination before the transplant operation, he was stable with no current mood or psychotic symptoms. His cognitive function was normal, with an MMSE score of 29. His valproate level was in the therapeutic range, and liver-associated enzymes were normal. He was able to fully understand the issues of renal transplantation and underwent an uncomplicated renal transplantation 1 month later. His posttransplant immunosuppressants included mycophenolate mofetil 500 mg twice daily and sirolimus 4 mg daily.

He did well for approximately 6 months on stable dosages of medications, during which time he secured his own apartment while continuing to use his sister's family as a source of social support. However, he then noted the subacute onset of decreased sleep, racing thoughts, impulsivity, and irritability. He had a minor motor vehicle accident while driving during the incipient manic episode. He was briefly admitted to a psychiatric hospital where his divalproex sodium was increased to 1,500 mg at bedtime, and he received a brief course of haloperidol. In subsequent clinical follow-up, he was given risperidone 1 mg orally at bedtime to help maintain a normal sleep pattern and to serve as prophylaxis against recurrent manic episodes. In the subsequent months he did well with mood stability and was able to return to work in customer service.

◆ **Diagnosis: Axis I—Bipolar I Disorder, Most Recent Episode Manic, Severe With Psychotic Features, 296.44; Adverse Effects of Medication Not Otherwise Specified, 995.2**

The therapeutic use of lithium may be associated with chronic renal insufficiency and eventual renal failure, which may eventually require dialysis and lead to the consideration of renal transplantation. In addition to the "usual" level of psychological adjustment required of the organ recipient in transplant surgery (receiving an organ from another, committing to lifelong immunosuppressants and close clinical follow-up, and the emotional aspects of receiving a kidney from a relative donor), patients with bipolar disorder may be prone to recurrent mood symptoms in the context of the stressors of these adjustments.

Patients who face renal failure from the use of lithium may approach this medical complication with significant ambivalence: anger that their compliance with a psychotropic medication has led them to needing an organ transplant operation, and the realization that one of the most effective psychotropic medications for their severe psychiatric illness is now unavailable to them for subsequent clinical need. The psychosomatic medicine care for these patients involves creative alternative psychopharmacology, assistance with adjustment to and assessment of psychiatric stability for candidacy for the transplant operation, and follow-up care in the posttransplant period.

References

Folstein MF, Folstein SE, McHugh PR: "Mini-Mental State": a practical method for grading the cognitive state of patients for the clinician. J Psychiatr Res 12:189–198, 1975

Kirby D, Ames D: Hyponatremia and serotonin re-uptake inhibitors in elderly people. Int J Geriatr Psychiatry 16:484–493, 2001

7

ENDOCRINE DISORDERS

Endocrinological disorders are intuitively interesting to psychosomatic medicine psychiatrists. These illnesses affect many metabolic systems and often have a significant psychiatric component to their classic symptom descriptions. Hyperthyroidism may present with elevated mood state or anxiety, whereas hypothyroidism may present with depression or cognitive impairment. In addition, treatments for endocrinological disorders (e.g., corticosteroids) may themselves be associated with psychiatric side effects. The patient with chronic endocrinological illness may have progressive loss of physical function from the complications of vascular disease and experience mood disturbance in this context. Toxic exposures in the form of suicide attempts may result in metabolic disturbances. Thus, the psychiatrist is well served by a stance of "thinking metabolically" when evaluating psychiatric illness in medically ill patients.

Paragangliomas, Depression, and Anxiety

A 42-year-old male travel writer was evaluated by the general medicine, endocrinology, and surgical services for clarification of treatment options for multiple paragangliomas (bilateral carotid body tumors and an abdominal paraganglioma at the bifurcation of the aorta). In the previous year he had learned that the abdominal paraganglioma was secreting excess catecholamines, as demonstrated by gradually increasing serum levels. Interestingly, he had no subjective awareness of any particular autonomic markers such as tachycardia or diaphoresis that served to herald catecholamine secretion. An avid runner, he followed his vital signs routinely and reported that his heart rate was commonly in the 60s and that he maintained a low-normal blood pressure without any other stigmata of catecholamine excess.

The patient was raised in a family with close-knit relationships with the extended family, who lived almost entirely in his hometown. He recalled that there were multiple individuals on his mother's side of the family who had depressive syndromes and variable anxiety. On his father's side, one uncle was a "hoarder" and had never agreed to evaluation or treatment. There was a strong family history of paragangliomas, but the patient was not certain if the individuals with known paragangliomas were the only ones with identified anxiety. Despite his experience with anxiety, he excelled academically and proceeded from college to graduate school in journalism. He confessed that secondary to his anxiety, he rarely attended classes in graduate school, recalling, for example, that he would become so preoccupied with finding the "correct route" to ride his bicycle to class that he would never make it to the building on time. During those years he increasingly relied on prescriptions for various benzodiazepines from multiple physicians to help ameliorate his anxiety. He took 65 mg of diazepam on the day he presented his master's thesis without any observed compromise of cognitive function. This proved to be a "wake-up call," and he sought medical assistance with gradual reduction and discontinuation of all benzodiazepines. He never experienced a panic attack and enjoyed extensive and remote travel. His avocation became his occupation as his travel writing gained increasing recognition.

In addition to his long history of anxiety, the patient reported two previous discrete episodes of major depression, both of which had gradually resolved within about 3 months of his family physician prescribing fluoxetine. Six weeks prior to his presentation with rising catecholamine levels, he had noticed the subtle onset of dysphoria accompanied by a loss of initiative and uncharacteristic diffidence. He found himself increasingly doubtful and inclined to draw negative conclusions about his abilities and worth. He felt guilty for having enjoyed his career, concluding that the pleasure he had derived from it demonstrated that it could not be virtuous. He had lost about 5 pounds, noticed that he was tightening his belt more than before, and complained about fragmented, unrestful sleep.

Mirtazapine 15 mg each evening was initiated and increased to 30 mg daily 2 weeks later after he had observed neither benefit (apart from better sleep) nor any autonomic findings such as elevated blood pressure, diaphoresis, headache, or tremor. He described a subsequent mild "numbing" or blunting of affect but also began to feel more hopeful and energized. Mirtazapine was increased to 45 mg nightly, and within the next week he experienced additional incremental improvement in outlook and mood, but not to the point of recapturing his baseline. Although content with the benefit he had achieved, he wished to know what other mood-enhancing agents could be considered if he had a future deterioration in mood.

◆ **Diagnosis: Axis I—Depressive Disorder Not Otherwise Specified, 311; Anxiety Disorder Not Otherwise Specified, 300.00**

This patient demonstrates the opportunity for lifelong learning. He presented with an unusual condition and surprised his multidisciplinary medical team by experiencing no autonomic consequences of his catecholamine excess. Furthermore, mirtazapine might not have been the psychiatry team's first choice given its noradrenergic activity. Surprisingly, it appeared to have had no effect on either his laboratory measures or his subjective experience.

Options for antidepressant augmentation without fear of aggravating catecholamine excess include lithium carbonate, triiodothyronine, modafinil, escitalopram, and low-dose atypical neuroleptic agents.

Alcohol Dependence and Isopropanol Poisoning: Mimicry of Metabolic Disease

A 53-year-old male with an unremarkable medical history other than known alcohol dependence was discovered unconscious in the restroom of the local bus station. In the emergency department, he was disoriented and combative. Laboratory tests included an unremarkable complete blood count apart from a mildly elevated mean corpuscular volume. His electrolytes were notable only for sodium of 132 mEq/L and potassium of 3.2 mEq/L. Liver enzymes were slightly elevated, with an aspartate aminotransferase of 109 U/L; troponin was negative. An arterial blood gas revealed a pH of 7.34, pO_2 of 94, pCO_2 of 37, and HCO_3 of 27. Ethanol and methanol levels were negative. However, isopropanol level was 1,002 µg/mL and acetone level was 2,071 µg/mL. Serum osmolality was 343 mOsm/kg, with a calculated serum osmolal gap of 64 mOsm/kg. A urine drug-abuse survey was positive only for ibuprofen and serum acetaminophen, and salicylate levels were negative.

The patient was admitted to a general medical service for management of isopropanol intoxication and was placed on one-to-one observation. Psychiatry was consulted to help assess whether the patient's ingestion of isopropyl alcohol was a suicide attempt. He reported leaving an alcohol treatment program prematurely 1 week earlier and proceeding to a local homeless shelter. Bereft of cash and unable to obtain further ethanol, he had consumed a bottle of rubbing alcohol (isopropanol). Although he gave an inconsistent account of depressive symptoms, he insisted he had no suicidal ideation. Instead, he emphasized a 35-year history of alcohol dependence with multiple treatment programs, one 7-year stretch of sobriety, and many relapses. He had had several medical hospitalizations for alcohol intoxication, including previous instances where he required intubation and observation in the intensive care unit.

The following morning, the patient ate breakfast, was fully oriented and appropriate during the medical team's rounds, and used the bathroom. Not long after returning to his bed, he became somnolent. Less than an hour later, his nurse was unable to awaken him. His vital signs were normal, but a wad of chewing tobacco was found in his mouth. Naloxone and flumazenil were administered intravenously with no response. He was transferred to the intensive care unit and required intubation. An emergent bronchoscopy revealed no abnormalities. Laboratory studies were notable for ethanol at 3,759 μg/mL, isopropanol at 455 μg/mL, and acetone at 753 μg/mL. A urine drug screening was positive only for ethanol.

The patient was extubated the following day and acknowledged having ingested an unknown quantity of hand sanitizer prior to his episode of unresponsiveness. The hand antiseptic available to the patient was 61% ethyl alcohol by weight in a 500-cc (16 fluid oz) pump bottle easily removed from a clasp holder mounted on the wall of his hospital room and at regular intervals in the hallway beyond his room. He was later discovered to have secreted yet another bottle of hand sanitizer in his pillowcase while still in the intensive care unit.

◆ **Diagnosis: Axis I—Alcohol Dependence, 303.90**

This patient provides several reminders to the clinician. A fruity odor may betray either isopropanol poisoning or diabetic ketoacidosis. Another distinct clue to his misuse of rubbing alcohol emerged with the calculated osmolal gap of 64 mOsm/kg. The normal range of the osmolal gap is approximately −10 to +10. A high osmolal gap reveals the presence of a low molecular weight substance that is osmotically active in the serum. The most common culprits are acetone (a metabolite of isopropanol and also present in diabetic ketoacidosis), ethanol, ethylene glycol, isopropanol, methanol, and mannitol. Treatment for isopropanol toxicity is hydration and conservative management. Another helpful prompt this patient affords is demonstration of the utility of a repeat drug screening in the face of an abrupt change in mental status, even in a hospitalized patient.

Alcohol-based hand sanitizers have become inescapable fixtures of hospital décor, liberally placed to facilitate efficient use by busy medical caregivers. This is an appropriate strategy to reduce transmission of infectious agents and is known to be more effective than soap-and-water hand washing, provided hands are not obviously soiled. It also takes less time and avoids the risk of recontamination from splashed water. Unfortunately, these agents are effective precisely because they typically contain isopropanol, *N*-propanol, ethanol, or some combination of these three. The solutions that contain more than 60% alcohol are the most effective.

Although there have been a handful of case reports describing intoxication from the ingestion of hand sanitizers, these have generally occurred in prisons or other higher-risk settings. However, as the alcohol content of these gels and solutions becomes increasingly well known, occurrence in the general hospital is likely to escalate unless consistent guidelines emerge regarding methods to reduce the risk of misuse.

Suggestions include placing the sanitizer in dispensers fixed to the wall and identifying additives to further reduce palatability. Until such measures are taken, psychosomatic medicine psychiatrists are well placed to raise awareness of this risk and, when working with patients such as this man, to advise the requesting service to remove alcohol-based hand sanitizers from the patient's room.

Psychosis and Acute Intermittent Porphyria

A 33-year-old Scandinavian woman with a history of gypsy-like wandering through a recurring cycle of Southern and Midwestern states announced to the emergency department receptionist that she had acute intermittent porphyria and had come for treatment because of increasing abdominal pain. She denied any prior occurrence of seizures or peripheral neuropathy but reported recurrent supraventricular tachycardia, vascular headaches, and previous episodes of depression. As she waited for medical evaluation, she clasped her arms together beneath her knees. Her knuckles blanched intermittently as she grimaced with evident pain. Between spasms of colicky abdominal pain, a nurse observed the patient making faces and watching her reflection in a stainless steel cabinet. She stared intently at the burnished surface. Although she was silent, her facial musculature swung like a pendulum from quizzical query to calming reply. She interrupted this wordless conversation to complain of nausea and to ask for an emesis basin.

When a resident physician asked to examine her, she volunteered, "You will not find a rash. People with acute intermittent porphyria do not get rashes. Your stethoscope can see many things but it will not hear me. I do not take medicines. They are too rich. You will not find them." The patient's blood pressure was mildly elevated and there was no questioning her abdominal pain, but the physical examination was nonspecific. Her urine drug screening was negative. She was admitted to the hematology service and intravenous hemin was initiated.

On her second hospital day, the patient confided to the housekeeping staff that she enjoyed living on the sixth floor of her mother's garage but she was especially grateful for the bicycle messenger who had arrived during the night to advise her not to defrost all the chickens she had just purchased from Wal-Mart. Her demeanor shifted abruptly and she asked the staff member to leave her room so she could sleep because "my son kept me awake the whole night with his earache."

The psychosomatic medicine psychiatry service was then consulted. The patient alluded to times of dysphoria and hopelessness and initially answered affirmatively to every question regarding neurovegetative signs and symptoms. Later, she denied each of these questions with equal certainty. When asked about command hallucinations, she replied "Do you mean when they tell me to hurt someone?" She then blandly disavowed such experiences. She acknowledged there were individuals about whom she had negative views, but she did not intend to harm them. Similarly, she yielded a history of past suicidal ideation but denied present suicidal intent. Soon thereafter, she volunteered that she experienced suicidal ideation with thoughts about shooting herself with a gun two or three times a week. She denied owning a gun and said she did not know anyone who owned a gun. When asked what dissuaded her from committing suicide, she said it was the thought of her son, but she then immediately added, "But not anymore…[because] a friend just called to tell me that my 6-year-old son passed away last night." She had spoken to her son that morning and when questioned about this she pointed to her head and said, "The problem's all here—maybe I don't know if he's dead."

When asked to interpret the proverb "People who live in glass houses shouldn't throw stones," she replied, "Don't look a gift horse in the mouth." The psychiatrist recounted the "Frank Jones story" with a monotonous tone and impassive expression: "Have I told you about my friend? His name is Frank Jones. His feet are so big that he has to put his pants on over his head." The patient smiled in response. When asked to explain her smile, she said, "I've seen the little guy do incredible things like the splits, so I suppose he probably could do that with his pants too, but it would be quite something." She paused, added that the size of Frank Jones' shoulders might create difficulties, and retreated to pensive silence.

The patient was fully oriented but when asked how long she had been in the hospital she said, "For 2 weeks, but I was discharged yesterday." When asked how it was possible that she had been discharged yet was still present, she mused, "Oh yeah, I guess I'm still here then." She was hypervigilant, snapping upright in bed whenever she heard her nurse walk past the door. She divulged paranoid ideation, whispering that, "People are trying to kill me with a gun." She knew this, she said, because multiple voices had disclosed this danger. Wary, she revealed that she had seen a number of unusual objects and events in her room, "like twisted pictures." She also described having the experience of holding an extended video clip of life in her fingers and watching, "the movie unwind."

The patient answered the same questions differently at various points in the interview and struggled with organizing her thoughts. It was difficult to establish whether she experienced psychotic thought content independent of the porphyria attacks. She initially said the voices faded but nonetheless remained in between episodes, but she later was emphatic that she only had "problems" when she had an exacerbation of porphyria. Previous medical records were sparse but supported the latter account. A year earlier, during a prior episode of acute porphyria, psychotic symptoms were initially treated with haloperidol, but the patient developed acute dystonia. Haloperidol was replaced by clonazepam and olanzapine with good results. The patient took both for several weeks but did not refill her prescription due to financial constraints. As far as could be determined, her psychotic symptoms had not earned notice until she returned to hospital with abdominal pain.

◆ **Diagnosis: Axis I—Psychotic Disorder Not Otherwise Specified, 298.9**

Acute intermittent porphyria is an autosomal dominant disease precipitated by defects in the enzyme porphobilinogen deaminase. As a consequence, the precursors of porphyrin, porphobilinogen and aminolevulinic acid, accumulate and cause neurological injury, although the mechanism of this damage is not understood. Abdominal pain, changes in mental status and other psychiatric symptoms, and peripheral neuropathies (more often motor than sensory) in the absence of a rash are common clinical findings.

Abdominal findings are commonly nonspecific despite the intensity of the pain. Nausea and vomiting are frequently observed, and patients often note an unusual history of constipation. Tachycardia and hypertension often accompany the acute attacks, and the latter may persist even after other physical symptoms have subsided. Neuropathies involve the lower extremities more commonly than the upper limbs. Depression and alterations in perception and mentation often attend acute attacks of intermittent porphyria.

Exhaustive lists of medications and other chemicals anecdotally or otherwise associated with attacks of porphyria exist, but they are not uniformly supported by consistent evidence. In sum, any substance or situation that provokes an increase in heme synthesis will boost the possibility of an acute attack in the 1%–2% of individuals with a known genetic defect who actually become symptomatic. Fasting and medications that are known to generate heightened P450 activity in the liver can trigger porphyria. More common culprits include alcohol, estrogen preparations, sulfonamides, and barbiturates.

Diabetes Mellitus Associated With Olanzapine

The metabolic burden of some atypical antipsychotic agents is central to the concerns about their use. Hyperlipidemia, weight gain, and diabetes mellitus may all be seen. When patients taking atypical antipsychotics present with acutely altered metabolism, the systemic and metabolic effects of these medications need to be jointly considered in the diagnosis and management.

Case 1

The patient was a 35-year-old woman with a history of bipolar disorder and no prior history of diabetes mellitus. She was started on olanzapine 10 mg at bedtime and valproate 500 mg three times daily for bipolar disorder after a manic episode. She initially tolerated this well, with improvement in her psychiatric symptoms. However, 3 months later, she was found to be unresponsive in her home. She had been complaining to family members of a 2-week period of polyuria, polydipsia, vomiting, fevers, and chills. She was transported to the emergency department, where she was unresponsive and diaphoretic and was discovered to be in acute hyperglycemic hyperosmolar nonketotic coma. Blood glucose was 1,896 mg/dL; other laboratory results included Na^+ of 161 mEq/dL, blood urea nitrogen of 55 mg/dL, creatinine level of 4.1 mg/dL, valproate level of 21 mg/L, and urine glucose of more than 1,000 mg/dL. The patient was admitted to the intensive care unit and treated with intravenous fluids, insulin drip, and antibiotics. Initially, her valproate and olanzapine were continued. After 9 days in the hospital, her blood glucose was 377 mg/dL despite large standing doses of insulin and increased doses from a sliding scale. A psychosomatic medicine consultation was then obtained.

On examination, the patient had a fluctuating level of consciousness, dysphoric affect, and no psychotic symptoms. Due to the connection between olanzapine and hyperglycemia, she was taken off of olanzapine while valproate was continued. After discontinuing olanzapine, her blood glucose level decreased to 149 mg/dL 3 days later. Her mood symptoms continued to be under control and her sensorium cleared. She was discharged in stable condition.

◆ **Diagnosis: Axis I—Bipolar Disorder Not Otherwise Specified, 296.80; Adverse Effects of Medication Not Otherwise Specified, 995.2**

Case 2

The patient was a 30-year-old schizophrenic man who had been treated with olanzapine 30 mg daily. He had no history of diabetes mellitus. He developed acute change in mental status after 2 days of vomiting of coffee grounds–colored emesis. On emergency evaluation, he was minimally responsive and in acute distress. Laboratory studies revealed hyperglycemia and pancreatitis, with a blood glucose level of 1,652 mg/dL, lipase of 2,172 U/L, and amylase of 638 U/L. Blood urea nitrogen and creatinine were 73 mg/dL and 5.6 mg/dL, respectively. Hemoglobin A_{1C} was 15.2%, and serum ketones were 80 mg/dL. Computed tomography revealed pancreatic inflammation and edema. He was admitted to the intensive care unit and given fluid resuscitation and an insulin drip. Olanzapine was stopped, and he received glyburide briefly; he required no further insulin or glyburide after 30 days. After a prolonged course in the hospital, he eventually recovered. His psychiatric symptoms were treated with aripiprazole 15 mg daily; aripiprazole was not associated with hyperglycemia. He was eventually discharged in stable condition.

◆ **Diagnosis: Axis I—Schizophrenia, Paranoid Type, 295.30; Adverse Effects of Medication Not Otherwise Specified, 995.2**

The connection between olanzapine and diabetes mellitus is increasingly being recognized in the clinical literature. For the psychosomatic medicine psychiatrist, the presentation of this complication in the general hospital is likely to be more dramatic and extreme than cases presenting in the psychiatry clinic. Extreme levels of hyperglycemia (as in the first case) may be associated with ketoacidosis. Once the patient's acute endocrinological issues are addressed, alternative psychotropic medications should be considered, with due concern of the risk of hyperglycemia from similar medications and the need for close monitoring of the endocrinological and psychiatric conditions in parallel. It is likely that olanzapine poses the greatest risk for atypical antipsychotic–associated hyperglycemia; however, the risk for hyperglycemia with clozapine, risperidone, and quetiapine is also significant. At this point, it appears that ziprasidone and aripiprazole may be less likely to be associated with hyperglycemia. In patients thought to represent significant risk for the development of diabetes mellitus (e.g., those with mild glucose intolerance or obesity), the psychosomatic medicine psychiatrist may need to modify the choice of antipsychotic medication.

Diabetes Mellitus, Diabetic Complications, and Depression

Diabetes mellitus is the prototype for metabolic disease with a high degree of psychiatric comorbidity. Indeed, depression is quite common in these patients. Whether attributable to psychodynamic factors (e.g., the loss of the healthy self, compromise on life goals to accommodate illness and complications, redefining the self as an ill person) or to more "neural" causes (e.g., the higher incidence of vascular dementia in diabetic patients with vascular complications, the chronic pain from diabetic peripheral neuropathy), the psychological burden in diabetes is clear and profound. In addition, the insulin-dependent diabetic has ready access to a medication that can be used in suicide attempts by hypoglycemia. The psychosomatic medicine psychiatrist is frequently confronted with such patients. The physician may need to alter the interview approach, the psychotherapy stance, and psychopharmacological management to optimally manage these patients.

> The patient was a 30-year-old white man with a history of insulin-dependent diabetes since childhood. Psychosomatic medicine consultation was completed due to noncompliant behavior with outpatient care that had resulted in several inpatient admissions for diabetic ketoacidosis and dehydration, for which the patient required aggressive fluid resuscitation. As a result of his diabetes and its complications, the patient had been unable to work or to attend school consistently and had lost touch with his peer group. He had become sullen and depressed; when depressed, he was not motivated to self-manage his insulin and blood glucose testing.
>
> On interview, the patient had a significant sense of life having passed him by. He blamed his illness and by extension his physicians for his loss of social connection and social opportunities. He was irritably depressed, with mixed and inconsistent neurovegetative signs, some episodes of notably poor sleep, and loss of weight. He had previously been given sertraline for depression, but he complained of significant gastrointestinal symptoms and aggravation of his symptoms of gastroparesis and had discontinued the medication. Due to the gastroparesis, he had frequent episodes of nausea and vomiting, which exacerbated his fluid balance status. Significantly, he refused to restart sertraline "or any medication like it" due to the gastrointestinal symptoms.
>
> Because of his insomnia and weight loss and his previous intolerance of sertraline due to gastrointestinal symptoms, the patient was prescribed mirtazapine 15 mg orally at bedtime. Mirtazapine was chosen due to its sedative properties, its likelihood of stimulating his appetite, and its postsynaptic 5-HT$_3$ receptor blockade activity, which were likely to not exacerbate his excess gastrointestinal symptoms as had happened with sertraline. He was able to tolerate this medication well, with improved sleep, mood, and appetite. Notably, he did not have the same medication-related gastrointestinal symptoms he experienced with sertraline. He was able to verbalize a willingness to pursue outpatient care after his hospitalization.

♦ **Diagnosis: Axis I—Major Depressive Disorder (Chronic), Recurrent, Severe Without Psychotic Features, 296.33**

The care of the young adult type I diabetic patient represents a challenging biopsychosocial case to the psychosomatic medicine psychiatrist. The presentation of a devastating illness that requires active self-management is a particular challenge to the young patient who is developing autonomy in other ways only to be burdened with managing a life-threatening illness. As a result of illness and its complications, age-appropriate activities and opportunities may be sacrificed entirely or at least significantly compromised. Such patients may develop a sense of (often hostile) dependency on the medical system that sustains them, but the anger about their physical limitations may be reflected in passive-aggressive behavior such as noncompliance, rebellion against the constraints "imposed" by medical self-management, and the like. These episodes of regression and acting out are, of course, often followed by acute episodes of metabolic decompensation and the need for acute hospitalization, which only perpetuates the sense of hostile dependency already established in many cases.

The challenge for showing empathy in such cases is that one must acknowledge the injustice of the patient's having become diabetic "through no fault of your own" yet simultaneously help the patient accept and embrace the idea that "even though it is not your fault that you are diabetic, it is your responsibility to self-manage it." This apparent paradox may not be intuitively obvious to patients but may need to be explained and appropriately "framed" by the psychiatrist as an opportunity for personal empowerment.

Mood disorders, specifically depression, are commonly encountered in diabetic patients. Full treatment of mood disorders is a clinical imperative. Management of depression may enable the patient to work on the insight-related issues described earlier. In addition, diabetics who are also depressed will likely be even poorer at self-management. Hence, management of depression in diabetic patients is appropriately framed as an intervention to facilitate the overall medical care of the patient.

As complications proceed apace in severe diabetes mellitus, there may be a sense of betrayal and fear in the patient. "I have followed my glucose and self-administered insulin for years only to develop these complications" may be a familiar lament. With the news of another functional complication, the patient may become more depressed and (often briefly) "want to give up." Suicidality in diabetic patients must be treated very seriously, because these patients have access to lethal means—insulin—and are often quite knowledgeable about the doses adequate to produce significant hypoglycemia. Empathic understanding of the loss of function and sense of existential threat represented by progression of diabetes requires a medically informed psychotherapist with working knowledge of the medical aspects of the case.

8

ONCOLOGY

The psychosomatic medicine treatment of cancer patients, or psycho-oncology, has quickly become, like transplant psychiatry, a psychiatric "sub-subspecialty." Although relatively few psychosomatic medicine psychiatrists treat cancer patients exclusively, the care of cancer patients is an important part of the work of the psychosomatic medicine psychiatrist. Few clinical conditions challenge the diagnostic, psychotherapeutic, and psychopharmacological skills of the psychosomatic medicine psychiatrist as much as dealing with the psychiatric aspects of cancer.

At the diagnostic level, patients with cancer can present in myriad ways. Patients with primary central nervous system (CNS) disease or CNS metastases from a distant primary lesion may present with delirium and/or dementia. Therefore, the initial evaluation of altered mental status in a known cancer patient (either at initial cancer diagnosis or in an established cancer patient) needs to first be directed toward a full systemic evaluation. Obviously, neuroimaging is needed to attempt to identify metastatic disease that can be structurally located. In addition, cancer patients are prone to syndrome of inappropriate secretion of antidiuretic hormone (this risk is reported to be higher in cancers of the lung or CNS), other disordered electrolyte metabolism, and abnormal liver enzyme levels from hepatic metastases.

Even after apparent structural and metabolic complications referable to cancer have been ruled out, there remains the important issue of "borderland" psychiatric symptoms with possible dual attribution. Many cancer patients have insomnia, low energy, fatigue, poor appetite, weight loss, and other "constitutional" symptoms.

The psychosomatic medicine psychiatrist, after eliciting a history of these symptoms, must then make an important attributional decision. Are the symptoms the direct consequences of the cancer itself? Are these symptoms due to the effects of cancer interventions, such as chemotherapy, oncological surgery, or radiation treatment (or, indeed, a combination of these), or are they due to a cancer-related depression episode?

Even if the clinician attributes these symptoms to a cancer-related mood episode, one must not take the jaundiced view "Of course you are depressed; after all, you have a life-threatening illness" and thus decline to offer psychiatric treatment for the mood disorder. In cases in which there is significant ambiguity and/or overlap between the attributed causes, it is probably best to err on the side of psychopharmacological treatment rather than withhold it, because a robust response to antidepressants may increase the quality of life for these patients.

Psychopharmacology in Cancer Patients

When choosing antidepressant treatment for cancer patients, the side effect profile of the various antidepressants is more important than in many other illnesses. For example, although selective serotonin reuptake inhibitor–related side effects of mild and transient gastrointestinal distress are usually well tolerated by other systemically ill patients, they may be quite problematic in the cancer patient with nausea from either a primary gastrointestinal cancer or as a side effect of chemotherapy. In addition, the mild appetite suppression seen with selective serotonin reuptake inhibitors and bupropion (although welcome to many obese patients) may be quite unwelcome and counterproductive in the anorexic and "wasting" cancer patient. Many cancer patients have cancer-related chronic pain; thus, a noradrenergic antidepressant such as venlafaxine, duloxetine, or mirtazapine may be additionally beneficial. Cancer patients with severe insomnia and weight loss might be good candidates for mirtazapine, which increases appetite and promotes sleep. Finally, severely depressed cancer patients with associated profound fatigue may benefit from either bupropion (providing there is no seizure or bulimia history) or a psychostimulant.

Psychotherapy in Cancer Patients

The psychotherapy approach to cancer can be similarly nuanced and challenging. With the patient who is extremely distressed over a new diagnosis, the psychotherapy approach may need to focus on assessment and management of acute suicidality. Such patients initially may catastrophize and develop excess and often distorted despair and an acute sense of hopelessness. An empathic stance combined with gentle challenging and reframing of catastrophic cognitions, encouragement of increased knowledge about cancer interventions, and simultaneous mobilization of social supports is often helpful. An important aspect of this intervention is to fully mobilize the multidisciplinary care model of the cancer center model, if cancer care is to be delivered at such an institution. The cancer center model is notable for its "early and active" inclusion of social support structures. Once patients (and their families) are established in the cancer center model, the risk of social isolation may be significantly mitigated.

As the case progresses, the clinician is well advised to remain vigilant for the development of changes in mood over time. There may be a greater risk for depression episodes when clinical interventions do not go well, when there is the discovery of metastatic disease, when there are medical complications, or when other similarly "discontinuous" clinical experiences occur. Finally, when cancer progresses and the patient's life expectancy grows short, there is an opportunity for grief work, reconciliation of key interpersonal relationships, making decisions on end-of-life care preferences, and issues of one's legacy.

Pancreatic Cancer and Denial

A 54-year-old male with a history of diabetes mellitus type 2, hyperlipidemia, hypertension, and recurrent pancreatitis was admitted for a Whipple procedure following the discovery of pancreatic cancer. Six days postoperatively he experienced mounting difficulty with anxiety, particularly in anticipation of discharge from the hospital and the need to self-inject insulin. On the evening prior to his intended discharge, he became acutely anxious and then unresponsive, prompting a psychiatric consultation. By the time the psychiatrist arrived, acute medical contributions had been excluded, and he was again alert and responsive without notable sequelae.

The patient was a priest in a rural parish whose responsibilities were many, in part because he had extended himself in several community ventures beyond his formal religious duties. He vaguely acknowledged prior anxiety after an ill-defined "heart attack" in 1980 as well as two episodes that he preferred to characterize as "burnouts" in 1984 and 1993. He associated these with increasing anxiety secondary to headlong commitment to his parish work, to the point where he became unable to sleep and essentially collapsed in exhaustion. He recalled brief utilization of a medication to calm him in 1984 but revealed that after the episode in 1993, he had taken an unknown medication for 2 years. He also described severe anxiety following a cholecystectomy in 2006 and added that his anxiety was associated with confusion and feeling "terrified," although he did not report concomitant autonomic findings apart from diaphoresis and chills.

The patient was lying flat on his back in his hospital bed, staring at the ceiling. He offered brief eye contact, and his hand was tremulous when he extended his arm to shake hands. His demeanor and speech had a brittle tone, as if the determined nonchalance might shatter without warning. His thought processes were intermittently tangential, with no evidence of a formal thought disorder. His mood was obscured by his resolute face, but his insistence on looking anywhere but at the examiner, coupled with facial twitching, betrayed his anxiety. Cognition was grossly intact in terms of his capacity to follow the flow of conversation and offer answers to questions without deferring to a family member, but when more formally assessed, he had difficulty identifying the date. He was not able to do serial sevens but spelled a five-letter word backwards accurately. He registered three words but was unable to recall them several minutes later, substituting other words instead.

The patient rated his current level of anxiety as "0/10" and professed perplexity that anyone thought he might have been anxious during his stay in the hospital. Questions directed to invite him to speak of his experience and perception of the future in light of his new diagnosis were answered instead by comments about his concerns for the people in his parish and a recurring recitation about how he had always sought to "empower people—that's my ministry." He denied any experience of depression whatsoever and said he was full of hope, describing his cancer as "a new beginning." He denied passive or active suicidal ideation, noting instead that he had "always been positive and upbeat."

The patient's extended family shed helpful light. They revealed that the earlier "anxiety" and "burnout" described by the patient had all been recurrent major depressive episodes. They also shared that he had begun to demonstrate familiar neurovegetative signs and symptoms in the 2 months prior to his presentation with abdominal pain leading to the diagnosis of pancreatic carcinoma.

◆ **Diagnosis: Axis I—Major Depressive Disorder, Recurrent, Severe Without Psychotic Features, 296.33**

On additional discussions with this patient's family members, one brother volunteered that the patient had always been intent upon perceiving and portraying himself through the lens of his identity as a priest; he had approached the subject of his emotions with difficulty and did not readily disclose any personal issues to his family, let alone his parishioners. The psychiatrist introduced a candid discussion about whether priests are allowed to be human, but the patient was very reluctant to engage the subject. He provided an impressive demonstration of the defensive vigor of isolation of affect, intellectualization, and denial.

Adenocarcinoma and Refusal of Treatment

The consult request wasted no words: "Refusing XRT" (i.e., patient refuses radiation therapy). But the demographic data added an intriguing twist to what had looked to be a straightforward request to assess capacity: the patient was middle-aged, and there was no indication of developmental delay, paranoia, or previous traumatic brain injury. In fact, the patient was a polite 53-year-old gentleman who acknowledged intermittent abdominal discomfort for the past 6 years. Infrequent and unrevealing evaluations suggested irritable bowel syndrome. A computed tomography (CT) scan had been recommended previously but was declined by the patient.

Two years prior to admission, the discomfort had become less crampy, but he attached no significance to this detail at the time. Over the previous 9 months, the lower-quadrant tenderness had become more persistent. He estimated having unintentionally lost approximately 20 pounds in the 6 months before recent episodic abdominal distension and profound fatigue brought him to the emergency department. He had no nausea, vomiting, or other symptoms suggestive of recurring bowel obstruction. In retrospect, he reluctantly affirmed that the character of his bowel movements had changed, but he seemed reluctant to discuss specifics and dismissed closer questioning by saying it was not the sort of detail to which he paid attention.

The emergency department physician obtained an abdominal and pelvic CT scan that revealed an extensive abdominal tumor with two areas of more discrete tumor present in the descending colon and rectal area. The patient consented to exploratory laparotomy and underwent a left colon resection with colostomy and omentectomy. The effort to debulk the tumor was suboptimal due to extensive involvement. Pathology was consistent with adenocarcinoma of the colon. Several mesenteric nodules were removed, and all were consistent with metastatic disease, but none of the 31 lymph nodes were positive for metastatic disease. Apart from a clostridial infection, the patient did well postoperatively. Persistent diarrhea despite a negative repeat test for *Clostridium difficile* toxin eventually yielded a diagnosis of lactase insufficiency. Medical oncology met with the patient to discuss various strategies for subsequent treatment. However, when radiation therapy was mentioned, the patient abruptly ended the conversation, firmly informed the consulting physician that he would have no part of radiation, and asked his primary team how soon he would be able to be sent home.

The psychiatry consultant was regarded with courteous but guarded interest. The patient acknowledged that his primary team had advised him of the forthcoming assessment and then volunteered that his principal psychiatric concern was mild ruminative anxiety, which was most prominent at night and the likely cause of his insomnia. He noted that it had been several nights since his last restful sleep because he had recently been preoccupied in the evenings with the fact that he was single and had limited resources at home to help manage the anticipated difficulties his new diagnosis would introduce. The patient described a dysphoric mood and associated symptoms that included insomnia, negative musing on the consequences of his surgery and diagnosis, diminished initiative, motivation, and energy, limited appetite, and concern for the future. His denial of suicidal ideation was both thoughtful and straightforward. He said he did not see himself as depressed, reiterated his hope for something to help with sleep, and thanked the psychiatrist as if to bring the interview to a conclusion.

The psychiatrist addressed this concern before proceeding to explain that the patient's dismissal of the oncology consultant had aroused the surgical team's concern that the patient might have lost his capacity for informed decision making. The patient stiffened, drew himself up defensively in bed, and replied, "The fact that I will not have radiation treatments is not a psychiatric issue! That's between me and my doctor, and I said, 'No.' There's nothing more to discuss. It is my choice, isn't it?" Attempts to approach this issue from different angles were unsuccessful. Eventually, the psychiatrist relented and, attempting to patch a ruptured sense of rapport, turned to more *pro forma* questions in anticipation of dictating the consultation note. It was only in seeking to round out his knowledge of the patient's developmental history that he stumbled upon the root of this man's unbending opposition to radiation therapy.

Probing for a less contentious path, the psychiatrist asked about the patient's hometown, intersecting highways, and how the county seat had grown over the years. One thing led to another as the physician listened and unobtrusively sketched the boundaries of the patient's youth. Adolescence was uneventful; young adulthood was not. Financial pressures on the family farm had magnified the differences between an energetic but sometimes impulsive young man and a wearying but wiser father. Back and forth they argued, each straining to oblige the other to see every issue from a different perspective. They wrestled and fought over decisions large and small, but never at the cost of failing to do each day's work well.

"He was a bull," said the patient wistfully. "Bull Meacham. Did you ever see *The Great Santini?* My pop didn't spend a day in the military but he could have been Bull Meacham. Yea, Pop was a bull."

"Was?" asked the psychiatrist. That is when the story unfolded, so painfully and gracefully that the psychiatrist wondered whether the patient realized he had become a guide, leading the physician through the labyrinth of his memory and unspoken grief.

The story was simple enough. The patient and his father had grown to respect one another and then to affectionately play to one another's strengths. The farm prospered. The patient's father was bothered by periodic abdominal pain, but the demands of the corn and cattle pushed complaining aside. His stamina flickered, and his suspenders became a necessity as his girth contracted. A storm system was forecast to settle in for 2 or 3 days with the promise of drenching the earth; there was still corn to come in and the patient and his father worked late into the night, halogen bulbs raising line upon line of corn stalk shadows awaiting the reaper. They paused for iced tea and his father leaned against the tractor tires, using the tread to scratch an elusive spot just between his shoulder blades. Then he doubled over in pain, slid to the ground and collapsed.

The doctor described the surgery, put a scan on the light box, outlined contrasting grays and blacks, and sat down. He recommended radiation therapy. It sounded straightforward and clean. The father could expect to experience fatigue and maybe diarrhea. One week after starting the daily radiation treatments, the patient's father was dead. The whole world slowed down and changed color. A blood clot, they said, but the patient had always known somewhere inside that it was the radiation. "I'm not making the same mistake Pop did," the patient said, to no one in particular.

◆ **Diagnosis: Axis II—V71.09, No Diagnosis**

One of the pleasures of consultation psychiatry is that no two consultations are ever alike. No two patients arrive at the intersection of medical illness and psychiatric evaluation with the same story. For some, the answer to the question may lie hidden in laboratory values. For another, the solution to the riddle may emerge only when a careful timeline is constructed. The patient who reflexively refused radiation therapy perceived no psychiatric quandary, whereas the psychiatrist saw no easy way through the thicket of resistance to even discuss the issue. Methodical discipline uncovered the answer.

Cross-Cultural and Language/Interpreter Issues in Breast Cancer and Pulmonary Emboli

A 65-year-old widowed Saudi Arabian woman presented with a right breast mass, a 5×5 cm open, purulent wound, and palpable bilateral axillary adenopathy. The patient complained of progressive fatigue, chronic cough, and midthoracic spine pain for the past 2 months. She spoke no English whatsoever, but her son, who was educated in Great Britain and spoke flawless English, accompanied her and firmly declined a professional interpreter, serving this station himself.

The patient described experiencing a burn to the right breast 3 years earlier, after which she noted subcutaneous nodules followed by open ulceration. She successfully hid this development until her family noted bleeding through her clothing. The patient also described having cared for her daughter who had died of metastatic breast cancer at the age of 30, 7 years earlier.

Her son said the patient had been advised that she did not have "cancer" but rather an "infection" and that he wished to tell her of her actual diagnosis privately later. The oncologist agreed, but emphasized that the patient needed to be told within the coming week so that she could make an informed decision regarding treatment. It subsequently became evident that the son did not inform the patient of her actual diagnosis. When confronted, he remained adamant that she only be told that she had an "infection."

Incisional biopsy confirmed an invasive Grade III/III ductal adenocarcinoma with positive estrogen and progesterone receptors.

Further evaluation revealed multiple left and right lung nodules suggestive of metastases, but no evidence of hepatic metastases. Lytic lesions of the thoracic spine were confirmed. The patient was placed on tamoxifen, and her adenopathy improved for several months. However, she began to experience rib pain and discontinued the tamoxifen, believing it to be responsible for her pain, increasing dyspnea, and nausea.

The patient returned from Saudi Arabia 1 year after her initial presentation complaining of dyspnea, diminished appetite, loss of energy, and a recurrent experience of chest heaviness. She was admitted to the hospital, and chemotherapy was initiated. An electrocardiogram indicated coronary ischemia, prompting an echocardiogram that revealed a mild pericardial effusion. An adenosine sestamibi scan indicated reversible ischemia, and the patient consented to a coronary angiogram. The angiogram demonstrated two small highly stenotic vessels, best managed medically rather than surgically.

At this point, the patient's complaints of dyspnea increased, and a right lower extremity deep venous thrombosis was found. She refused a CT Imatron scan and other diagnostic tests proposed to evaluate the possibility of a pulmonary embolus. The intensive care team elected to heparinize the patient, but when the intravenous team approached, the patient repeatedly held up her hands as if to say, "Stop!" and would not allow the intravenous line to be placed. The patient's son insisted that his mother be treated, stating, "She is out of her mind and has no idea what she is saying when she refuses. You must treat her." Nursing staff had observed no evidence of delirium; to the contrary, the patient had been alert throughout the day and appeared to track events in her room appropriately. She had also been speaking with her son throughout the day, and he had not expressed any previous concern about confusion.

At 11:00 on a Friday evening, psychiatry was consulted to assess the patient's capacity to make an informed decision regarding her refusal of intravenous placement for heparin therapy. However, the patient's son planted himself in front of her room and announced, "In my country, the family makes the decision for the patient. I am the oldest son, and I insist that my mother be treated. Pay no attention to her protests; she is confused."

Upon arrival of the Arabic interpreter, the psychiatric consultant approached the patient's son and again sought permission to proceed. The son replied that he alone would be his mother's interpreter and that he would not allow the interpreter to be in the room, even as an observer. Following considerable discussion, he stated that his opposition was grounded in the fear that his mother would learn her true medical diagnosis. "I know you people," he said, "you refuse to tell lies, and she will learn the truth from you one way or another. She is a very intelligent woman, and she will learn the truth." He reiterated his offer to serve as the interpreter, stating, "Let me lie for you so that you do not have to lie."

The psychiatrist clarified that the immediate goal was to assess the patient's decision-making capacity and that this could be accomplished without intruding upon the agreement that the son claimed he had reached with the patient's primary oncologist (a claim later discovered to be spurious)—that is, to withhold the diagnosis of cancer from the patient. The son was dubious of this offer, made a few references to intended legal action if his mother learned her actual diagnosis, and reiterated that he alone would serve as her interpreter. When the psychiatrist responded that an objective consultation could only be performed with the assistance of the interpreter, the son replied, "There is no need for further assessment because I can guarantee that my mother will not refuse any further treatment."

◆ Diagnosis: Axis I—Acculturation Problem, V62.4

This case illustrates a collision of cultural values and priorities that increasingly accompanies the mobility and porous boundaries of modern international medical care. Unable to express herself in English, the patient presented for care knowing only what her family had elected to tell her and whatever her own experience and counsel suggested. Her prior role as caretaker for her daughter during the daughter's progressive consumption by cancer surely cast her own acquaintance with illness in a more informed light. Nonetheless, she had traveled around the world to receive care that was unavailable at home but was now being deliberately described for her in terms that could only have come from home (i.e., "infection" and "antibiotic"). Deprived of a fuller accounting of her disease, its treatment, and prognosis, she later concluded that symptoms of metastatic bony involvement must be the product of her treatment and unwittingly joined forces with her cancer by discontinuing tamoxifen.

Back in the United States for further assessment and treatment, she had no way of knowing the earnest discussions she provoked as various physicians and medical caregivers wrestled with how to integrate respect for the son's interpretation of their cultural values with a more Western emphasis on the covenantal sanctity of the patient–physician relationship. This separation was strenuously maintained by the son's false report to the hospital team that the patient's outpatient oncologist had agreed not to inform her of her diagnosis and was further extended by his unwillingness to allow an independent interpreter within earshot of his mother.

Neurologic Paraneoplastic Syndrome and Renal Cell Carcinoma

A 64-year-old female Jehovah's Witness experienced the sudden onset of aphasia, right facial paralysis, and left extremity weakness. These symptoms resolved entirely over 3 hours, and a brain magnetic resonance imaging scan and magnetic resonance angiogram (MRI/MRA) and transthoracic echocardiogram (TTE) were normal. Three months later she had recurrence of the aphasia and weakness that again resolved completely. Within days, however, the aphasia recurred and progressively worsened. A head CT scan and carotid ultrasound were normal; a repeat MRI/MRA was again unremarkable. A second TTE revealed a patent foramen ovale, and warfarin was begun. An electroencephalogram showed mild nonspecific generalized slowing.

Months later, the patient had a generalized tonic/clonic seizure that resulted in hospitalization. Examination revealed significant cognitive impairment limiting the neuropsychological assessment. The only neurological findings included diffuse hyperreflexia, bilateral Hoffman's sign, and a Babinski sign on the left. Her condition worsened as her level of alertness and speech deteriorated. She displayed grabbing behaviors and spontaneous unintelligible speech suggestive of visual and auditory hallucinations. Her coordination, muscle tone, and gait characteristics waxed and waned. She displayed prominent grasp, snout, and glabellar reflexes. The remainder of the physical examination was unremarkable.

Laboratory assessment revealed an elevated sedimentation rate of 110 mm/hour (normal rate is <29), low hemoglobin of 11.4 g/dL (normal, 12.0–15.5), sodium of 128 mEq/L (normal, 135–145), alkaline phosphatase of 547 U/L (normal, 108–282), γ-glutamyltransferase (γ-GT) of 373 U/L (normal, 6–29), and alanine aminotransferase (ALT) of 159 U/L (normal, 9–29). Urinalysis and urine cytology were negative. The remainder of her laboratory assessment was unremarkable and included immunoglobulin G and M (IgG and IgM) phospholipid antibodies, a paraneoplastic autoimmune panel consisting of assays for acetylcholine receptor–binding antibody (AChR-binding Ab), antineuronal nuclear antibody (ANNA-I or anti-Hu), ANNA-2 (anti-Ri), Purkinje cell cytoplasmic autoantibodies–1 (PCA-1) (anti-Yo), amphiphysin, striated muscle antibody, N-type calcium-channel binding antibody, P/Q-type calcium-channel binding antibody, and a rheumatologic panel consisting of cryoglobulins, cryofibrinogen, anti-S DNA, rheumatoid factor, rapid plasma reagin (RPR), cytoplasmic-staining and perinuclear-staining antineutrophil cytoplasmic antibodies (ANCA), antinuclear antibody (ANA)–2 cascade, and an extractable nuclear antigen (ENA) antibody scan.

An electroencephalogram revealed generalized slowing consistent with delirium. Cerebrospinal fluid examination revealed mild elevation of albumin at 54.3 mg/dL (normal, 0–27.0), total nucleated cell count was six mononuclear cells per milliliter (normal, <5). Cytology studies, assays for neuron-specific enolase, and polymerase chain reaction for *T. Whippleii* were unremarkable. An MRI of the head, with and without gadolinium, showed minimal meningeal enhancement over both convexities. A cerebral angiogram did not display evidence of vasculitic inflammation.

Although the patient's initial urinalysis and urine cytology were unremarkable, her anemia worsened and a subsequent peripheral blood smear revealed abnormal red blood cell morphology with mild acanthosis, red blood cell stippling, poikilocytosis, and anisocytosis, all of which suggested possible renal disease. An ultrasound of her lower abdomen and pelvis showed a 3-cm solid mass in the left upper quadrant that appeared to be arising from the mid-upper pole of the left kidney. A CT scan confirmed this lesion to be a 5-cm heterogeneous enhancing solid mass with cystic degeneration seen in the left lateral mid-kidney, consistent with renal cell carcinoma. There was no obvious evidence of tumor spread.

The patient's delirium rendered her incapable of understanding her situation or making any treatment decisions. Her husband, in concert with her children, made the decision to proceed with a nephrectomy. He was advised of the likely requirement for blood transfusion and the risk of increased morbidity without access to such support. After further careful deliberation, the family concluded that the patient would prefer to honor her religious beliefs and forgo transfusion. The initial surgical team was unwilling to proceed under these circumstances. Eventually, with the assistance of the patient's religious community, a surgical group with deliberate experience in providing medical care to Jehovah's Witnesses without the use of blood transfusions was located, and the patient was transferred to their institution.

With the aid of an artificial blood substitute, the patient underwent radical nephrectomy without complication. Surgical pathology confirmed the presence of renal cell carcinoma. Clarity of

mental status and motor strength improved dramatically after nephrectomy. Within 3 months she had returned to her premorbid
level of function. Two years later, she had no recollection of her extended delirium but was otherwise doing well and functioning normally in her daily life.

◆ **Diagnosis: Axis I—Delirium, 293.0**

Cancer precipitates neurological and psychiatric manifestations
by direct metastasis or through metabolic, vascular/embolic, nutritional, infectious, or ischemic processes resulting from tumor inva-
sion of vital organs or occurring as treatment side effects. Much less
commonly, cancer causes neuropsychiatric symptoms via autoimmune mechanisms, thought to be mediated by specific antineuronal
antibodies.

This diverse group of disorders composes the neurologic paraneoplastic syndromes (NPS). Signs and symptoms vary widely, making the diagnosis difficult. Moreover, NPS can present in a variety of
fashions. Paraneoplastic cerebellar degeneration, paraneoplastic
myoclonus-opsoclonus, cancer-associated retinopathy, motor neuron disease, Lambert-Eaton myasthenic syndrome, and stiff-man
syndrome and paraneoplastic encephalomyelitis (PEM) have been
described. Prognosis of NPS is generally poor. Outcomes often include long-term neurological deficits or death. This patient's experience illustrates the dramatic effect early treatment can have, and
thus the importance of accurate diagnosis.

PEM itself may manifest as discrete syndromes such as, in order of
decreasing frequency, sensory neuropathy, limbic encephalitis, brain
stem encephalitis, motor neuron dysfunction, and autonomic dysfunction, depending on the areas and extent of CNS involvement.
More commonly, however, there is multifocal involvement of the
CNS with mixed symptoms. The entities classified under PEM
share common pathological findings and may share the presence of
the neuron-specific antigen anti-Hu (ANNA-1).

The clinical diagnosis of PEM is elusive. Electroencephalographic
results are often initially normal but later show nonspecific slowing
consistent with delirium, similar to that detected in this patient. CT
and MRI are frequently unrevealing, although there are reports of
observed signal changes in a variety of brain areas: the limbic regions,

medial temporal lobes, amygdaloid nuclei, and hypothalamus. The diagnosis of PEM can be made with certainty when tissue specimen reveals the characteristic histopathological features of neuronal cell loss, astrocytic gliosis, microglial proliferation, and perivascular infiltration. The diagnosis of limbic encephalitis is made when limbic involvement is predominant. Limbic encephalitis is the second most common type of PEM and is a well-described paraneoplastic syndrome characterized by a triad of memory loss, affective symptoms, and seizures, all of which were present in this patient.

In the absence of a histopathological examination, PEM can be diagnosed when anti-Hu antibodies are present in the serum. The antibodies that have been described in association with NPS seem to be specific to a certain type of tumor as well as the particular clinical neurologic paraneoplastic syndrome.

Growing evidence exists for the presence of other unnamed proteins, such as one found in the serum of patients with stiff-man syndrome. Frequently, however, patients who have NPS either do not have demonstrable antineuronal antibodies or may have atypical antibodies that are not detected in commercially available assays. Whether these are entities that exist separately from antibody-positive syndromes is controversial. Some patients may have high titers of autoantibodies and yet never develop a demonstrable tumor. On the other hand, as with this patient, some individuals with clinical PEM have no detectable autoantibodies.

Numerous tumors are associated with NPS. A review of the literature reveals that PEM alone has been associated most commonly with small-cell lung cancer. However, testicular cancer, ovarian cancer, Hodgkin's disease, and breast, gastric, uterine, and colon tumors have also been associated with PEM. Renal cell carcinoma is much less common.

Prognosis for limbic encephalitis specifically, and NPS generally, is poor, but some reports exist of reversal of the neuropsychiatric symptoms after treatment of the cancer, especially renal cell cancer. Although lung and ovarian cancers are the most common causes of NPS, renal cell carcinoma should be considered. When renal cell carcinoma is the underlying cause of NPS, autoantibodies that are frequently associated with NPS from other cancers may not be present.

Malignant Melanoma, Stages of Grief, and Coping

A 28-year-old white woman with a history of stage 4 metastatic malignant melanoma presented to the emergency department of a university medical center with an episode of hematemesis at home; this was followed by another episode of hematemesis in the emergency department. The patient also had daily episodes of melena for 1 month prior to presentation to the emergency department. She was admitted to the internal medicine service with an upper gastrointestinal bleed, believed to be secondary to the use of nonsteroidal anti-inflammatory drugs and alcohol. An internal medicine resident, concerned that he had found multiple bruises and lacerations on the patient's knuckles that she had acquired during a drunken "wall punching contest," requested a psychiatry consultation for assessment of suicidality and alcohol dependence.

The patient had been diagnosed with malignant melanoma at age 16, which after initial treatment appeared to have been in clinical remission until she developed a small bowel obstruction due to a recurrence of the melanoma at age 28. She required two bowel surgeries for cancer recurrence within 3 months, the last operation having been 5 months prior to her current presentation. The patient was found to be at stage IV, and at this stage "prognosis for long-term survival is poor, with 1-year survival rates ranging from 41–59%" (Balch et al. 2001). She had been advised by her oncologist not to get pregnant.

On initial psychiatric interview, the patient was quite open about describing her reckless behavior. She reported drinking alcohol to the point where she felt "out of control" and depended on others to care for her. She had been drinking almost daily, typically five drinks of hard liquor a day, for several years. She often began her day with a beer. She had also used methamphetamine in the past but had stopped 7 years prior to her current presentation. The patient described drinking alcohol with a group of male friends, who would then compete in various contests such as "wall-punching." She had sustained multiple bruises as a result of having fallen down while intoxicated.

The patient denied ever purposefully intending to harm herself and did not take part in self-damaging activities when sober. She recognized that she had a problem with "co-dependency" but felt that although her alcohol use resulted in dangerous behavior, she could stop drinking whenever she wanted. She was followed by a community psychiatrist via telephone visits and had been prescribed lamotrigine 300 mg daily and sertraline 100 mg daily for bipolar disorder. She also had a psychotherapist whom she had been seeing "as needed" since her cancer diagnosis at age 16. The patient felt that she had coped well with her initial cancer diagnosis by "remaining optimistic" and actively engaging in treatment, noting that she had already "proven the doctors wrong" by being in remission for more than 10 years. She denied any significant concern over her recent cancer recurrence.

The consulting psychosomatic medicine psychiatrist encouraged the patient to consider the negative consequences of her drinking and to reengage with her psychotherapist for more frequent follow-up. A subsequent upper gastrointestinal endoscopy revealed no active bleeding, and the patient was discharged to home on a proton pump inhibitor and her outpatient psychotropic medications.

◆ **Diagnosis: Axis I—Bipolar Disorder Not Otherwise Specified, 296.80; Alcohol Dependence, 303.90; Axis II— Dependent Traits, Rule Out Dependent Personality Disorder, 301.6**

This case of a young woman diagnosed with a malignant melanoma in her teens demonstrates the multiple potential psychiatric issues that can arise when normal psychological development is challenged by serious medical illness and when recurrence further threatens longevity. Although many factors play a role in the formation of personality and coping style, this patient's psychosocial development likely took a turn when she was first diagnosed with melanoma at age 16. Normal adolescence is a time for adjustment as teens vie for greater independence and a sense of individuality, and the diagnosis of serious illness may thrust adolescents back to an earlier stage of psychological development marked by greater dependency. For this patient, although dependency may have served as a fairly effective coping strategy during the initial cancer treatment, its continued use has proven maladaptive in later adolescence and adulthood. The patient admitted to continued high levels of "co-dependency" in adult relationships that she consciously perpetuated via frequent substance abuse.

Kübler-Ross (1973) wrote about the stages of grief typically encountered in persons experiencing a great loss or life change. Briefly, the stages in usual order of appearance (with typical reactions to the impending loss) are

◆ *Denial:* The initial stage: "It can't be happening."
◆ *Anger:* "Why me? It's not fair."

+ *Bargaining:* "Just let me live to see my children graduate."
+ *Depression:* "I'm so sad, why bother with anything?"
+ *Acceptance:* "It's going to be OK."

Individuals are not necessarily expected to go through all stages or to conform to the suggested order; however, successful resolution of the stages may lead to a greater sense of comfort and security for people facing a loss.

Our patient's reaction to her recurrence of cancer at age 28 continued to fluctuate between denial and anger, evidenced by her inability to address the seriousness of her illness while sober and her self-directed and self-destructive rage while intoxicated. It remained unclear whether the personality pathology, substance abuse, and mood disturbance seen in this patient would have occurred regardless of the early onset of life-threatening medical illness, but clearly this patient's ongoing experience and adjustment to cancer continued to be strongly affected by her adult psychopathology, preventing her from experiencing the typical stages of grief in an adaptive manner.

Research into the emotional and social adjustment of survivors of childhood cancer has yielded inconsistent findings as to the long-term effects. Although many studies have shown overall good psychological functioning in survivors of childhood cancer, others have shown specific problems related to education, work, marriage, and concerns about fertility (Langeveld et al. 2002). Survivors of childhood cancer may have higher rates of depression, alcoholism, suicide attempts, negative mood states, tension, anger, and confusion (Lansky et al. 1986; Zeltzer et al. 1997). Factors related to elevated risk of poor adjustment included older age at follow-up, greater number of cancer relapses, and severe functional impairment (Elkin et al. 1997; Langeveld et al. 2002).

This patient's cancer had been limited to her initial lesion and subsequent bowel metastases, and her current cancer treatment was limited to surgery; other factors that may further complicate the psychiatric symptomatology of oncological patients include disfigurement from oncological surgery, side effects from chemotherapy and radiation, metastatic involvement of the CNS, and various paraneoplastic syndromes. Psychotropic medication selection must be carefully thought out because of the many possible medication interactions and the hematopoietic side effects seen with several psycho-tropic medications. Psychotherapy focused on end-of-life issues may help patients effectively resolve barriers to acceptance and move on to other tasks such as saying goodbye.

Uterine Cancer, Bipolar Disorder, and Delirium

A 78-year-old woman was diagnosed with stage IIIB endometrial can-cer after a total abdominal hysterectomy and bilateral salpingo-oo-pherectomy. She initially appeared to tolerate the surgical procedure well, except for some reluctance to get out of bed. She was discharged to a nursing home for rehabilitation but returned to the hospital 23 days after the surgery for wound dehiscence and "failure to thrive." Since admission to the nursing home, the patient had stopped eating or getting out of bed. The psychosomatic medicine service was con-sulted for depression and to rule out suicidal ideation.

Although the stage IIIB 1-year survival for uterine cancer is esti-mated at 70.6%, 3-year at 51.7%, and 5-year survival at 30.2% (Creasman et al. 2003), the patient was quite certain that her diag-nosis meant imminent death. She had been living on a ranch with her 80-year-old female partner (who was blind) and thought she would never be able to return to the active lifestyle she had enjoyed. The patient reported having consented to the cancer surgery, which she had not expected to survive, for the benefit of her son and grandchil-dren. The patient's son revealed that prior to surgery, before the pa-tient even knew the extent of her cancer and her prognosis, she had encouraged her partner to join her in a mutual suicide pact.

On mental status examination the patient was alert with a fair level of engagement, depressed mood, and mildly restricted affect. She was motorically slowed and endorsed a number of neurovege-tative symptoms; her Mini-Mental State Examination (MMSE; Fol-stein et al. 1975) score was 26. The patient recalled several prior episodes of depression characterized by anhedonia, low energy, and poor motivation. She had taken fluoxetine (unknown dosage) during one depressive episode but noted that it had "stopped working" after 6 months of treatment. The patient's family history was significant for a sister who had received electroconvulsive therapy (ECT) for depression, with resultant memory loss; a grandfather who was in-stitutionalized for an unknown psychiatric illness; and a cousin who had killed his parents in consequence of the symptoms of an un-known psychiatric illness.

She received a diagnosis of major depression, severe, and mirtaza-pine was started for depression, anorexia, and insomnia. Mirtazapine was started at 7.5 mg nightly and increased to 15 mg several days later. Within a few days of treatment, the patient was irritable and labile, with increased energy and impulsive acting-out behavior. A 24-hour bedside sitter was recommended for active thoughts of suicide. Collateral sources revealed prior episodes of mood lability with increased goal-directed activity and decreased need for sleep. Her diagnosis was revised to bipolar disorder, most recent episode depressed, severe, and she was prescribed valproic acid extended release, which was titrated over 2 weeks to a dosage of 1,000 mg at night.

During the next several weeks, the patient became more resistant to medical treatment and refused tube feeds, physical therapy, and intravenous line placement. The psychosomatic medicine service was asked to evaluate the patient's decisional capacity to refuse these interventions. Attempts made by the treating psychiatrists to engage the patient in discussion about her expectations for the future were met with resistance in the form of sarcasm and morbid humor. She was found lacking in decisional capacity due to poor appreciation of her prognosis and growing paranoid delusions regarding hospital personnel (once accusing them of feeding her a meal saved from the prior week). Her son acted as decision-maker surrogate.

She then became delirious, with waxing and waning level of consciousness, visual hallucinations, and attentional deficits. The patient was found to have elevated serum ammonia of 81 μmol/L. The psychosomatic medicine service then recommended discontinuation of valproic acid because of its likely contribution to the patient's delirium via hyperammonemia; lactulose was also given, and the patient's ammonia level subsequently decreased to 22 μmol/L. Quetiapine, initially 25 mg twice a day and titrated up to 50 mg twice a day, was added for its mood-stabilizing and antidelirium activity. The patient's son consented to various procedures including the introduction of a percutaneous endoscopic gastrostomy tube for feeds and a peripherally inserted central catheter line for intravenous access. The psychosomatic medicine team discussed ECT with the patient's son, who noted that his mother had years ago seen her sister develop memory deficits from ECT and had said that she would never want this treatment.

Mirtazapine (which had been continued after valproate was added) was stopped 5 weeks after initiation when the patient began the antibiotic linezolid for vancomycin-resistant enterococci urinary tract infection and methicillin-resistant *Staphylococcus aureus* pneumonia. Quetiapine was discontinued due to oversedation. Various other medications, including aripiprazole (initial dosage 10 mg/day in divided dosing, titrated to 15 mg/day), lamotrigine (25 mg/day), and donepezil (5 mg/day; case report data showing utility in opiate-related altered mental status [Slatkin and Rhiner 2004; Slatkin et al. 2001]) were prescribed for delirium and mood stabilization.

The patient had few lucid periods over her last few weeks of hospitalization, and during these times she continued to endorse feelings of depression and hopelessness. After long discussions with the primary team, the psychosomatic medicine service, and the patient's family, the patient was discharged to a skilled nursing facility on hospice care. She died 6 weeks after discharge.

◆ **Diagnosis: Axis I—Bipolar I Disorder, Most Recent Episode Depressed, Severe With Psychotic Features, 296.54; Delirium, 293.0**

This case presented a complicated array of ethical, medical, and psychological issues that were heavily debated among the many treating physicians on the case. Among the psychosomatic medicine topics relevant to this case were decisional capacity determinations (which can be particularly difficult when they involve refusal of medical treatment in serious illness), suicidality in the medically ill, and the difficulty in treating the depressive phase of bipolar disorder in a patient with multiple comorbidities.

Patients are generally assumed to have the ability to understand medical information and make well-reasoned decisions. The ethical principle of autonomy ensures that competent patients determine the course of their own medical care. However, in cases in which a patient's ability to make good decisions is compromised, physicians must turn to another ethical principle, that of beneficence, to ensure the interests of the impaired patient are served. Although the vast majority of decisional capacity determinations are informally conducted by providers offering various treatments, psychiatrists (especially psychosomatic medicine specialists) are often called upon to make recommendations when a patient's ability to give informed refusal or consent in unclear. The standards typically applied in assessing a patient's medical decisional capacity are based on Appelbaum and Grisso's (1988) model. To demonstrate decisional capacity, patients must be able to

1. Communicate a clear and consistent preference
2. Understand the risks, benefits, and alternatives to the proposed course of treatment

3. Appreciate the significance of the information given to them about their illness and proposed treatment
4. Rationally manipulate this information in order to compare and evaluate options

Applying this model, a psychosomatic medicine psychiatrist can effectively evaluate a patient's cognitive ability to make medical decisions and can identify illogical and psychotic thought processes that may impair decision making. Unfortunately, this model does not necessarily consider the impact of the patient's emotional state and the effect depression may have on medical decision making. Many serious illnesses are associated with increased rates of major depression (Cassem 1995), and depression can clearly alter patients' view of their lives, making many situations appear bleak and hopeless (Kleespies et al. 2000). We found this to be the case for our patient, who was certain that her cancer would be very quickly terminal despite contrary evidence in the literature.

Sullivan and Youngner (1994) pointed out that "determining whether someone with a serious (or especially, terminal) medical illness is competently assessing his or her quality of life can be exceedingly difficult." However, these writers, in reviewing the literature on the impact of depression on decisions regarding life-sustaining treatments, found mixed results regarding the impact of depression and its treatment on subject decisions (Sullivan and Youngner 1994).

Although psychosomatic medicine psychiatrists generally recommend that patients facing a serious illness adequately address depression before deciding to halt care, we do not often question their ability to make this decision. However, in the case of this patient, where depression was sufficiently severe to impair her appreciation of her prognosis and she was actively seeking ways to end her life, "refusal of care" was difficult to distinguish from "suicidality." Although writers have questioned whether this distinction is ethically meaningful (Brock 1992; Sullivan and Youngner 1994), it continued to be quite poignant to the consulting psychosomatic medicine psychiatrists because prevention of suicide is often a main focus of psychiatric care. In fact, the presence of suicidality in a psychiatric patient is generally considered evidence that the patient is incompetent to refuse needed psychiatric interventions, which, in effect, are intended to prolong life (Sullivan and Youngner 1994). To quote Sullivan and Youngner (1994) on this topic: "In psychiatry, when refusal of life-saving treatment occurs, the burden of proof concerning competence is on the patient who desires to die; in internal medicine, the burden of proof concerning competence is on the physician who wishes to override the patient's refusal." The decision to deprive the patient of her "autonomy" was not taken lightly and weighed as a heavy burden on all treatment team members and the patient's son. As the patient became delirious, her diminished capacity to make medical decisions was more apparent.

Regarding the treatment undertaken for the patient's depression, the presence of bipolar disorder, the emergence of an unusual medication side effect, and the potential for a dangerous drug–drug interaction converged to make psychopharmacological treatment quite challenging. Initial evaluation revealed only the presence of symptoms of major depression, and mirtazapine was started accordingly. This medication was chosen for its sedating and appetite-stimulating properties. Another advantage of mirtazapine in medically ill individuals is the relative lack of drug–drug interactions.

A rapid change in agitation levels following mirtazapine therapy prompted a more thorough examination of past psychiatric history from additional collateral data sources, revealing a history consistent with bipolar disorder. At this point, the decision was made to add a mood stabilizer (valproic acid), and mirtazapine was continued. The patient experienced increased serum ammonia, a reported side effect of valproic acid (Wadzinski et al. 2007), and this medication was stopped. The later introduction of the antimicrobial medication linezolid brought a halt to the use of mirtazapine. Linezolid, an antibiotic used for infection with resistant organisms, is a reversible monoamine oxidase inhibitor, and as a result it has the potential for causing serotonin syndrome when given in conjunction with antidepressants. In cases of severe depression, especially where medications are poorly tolerated or contraindicated, ECT is often a good option. Unfortunately, in this case, a family history of memory problems after ECT made this treatment unappealing to the patient's surrogate. The patient's discharge to hospice care likely represented the fulfillment of her initial desires; sadly, it was never clear if adequate treatment of her depression would have changed the outcome.

Carcinomatous Meningitis, Depression, Anxiety, and Delirium

The role of psychosomatic medicine psychiatry in comanagement of terminal cancer patients may integrate diagnosis of neuropsychiatric illness, management with medications, and assistance to patients and loved ones in dealing with impending death, existential despair, and final reconciliation of relationships.

The patient was a 54-year-old white man with a history of Hodgkin's disease (in remission for more than 20 years) who was admitted to the neurology service at a university medical center with relatively new onset and recently progressive unsteadiness of gait, dysarthria, facial weakness, lumbar back pain, and urinary hesitancy. These symptoms had been present for approximately 2 months and had rapidly escalated over the several weeks prior to admission. Neurological examination at admission revealed weakness of several cranial nerves as well as significant gait ataxia.

The patient had a history of mild anxiety disorder and depression and had been taking bupropion for a number of years with good effect prior to the onset of his physical symptoms. The psychosomatic medicine service was asked to evaluate the patient's worsening of anxiety and insomnia. At the time of initial consultation, the patient was awaiting definitive diagnosis of his new neurological illness, and he was very concerned that he had a recurrence of cancer.

On examination, the patient was notably restless and anxious. The presence of protective goggles (a cranial nerve deficit prevented him from closing his eyes) added to the patient's appearance of hypervigilance. He had sialorrhea and his speech was dysarthric, also due to cranial nerve involvement. His MMSE score was 29. Based on recommendations from the psychosomatic team, bupropion was tapered and discontinued and mirtazapine 15 mg nightly was started for depression, anxiety, and insomnia. The orally dissolving form of mirtazapine was chosen because of his dysphagia. Lorazepam was also given as needed for acute anxiety.

A chest CT showed a lung mass, and a lumbar puncture revealed the presence of carcinomatous meningitis, representing metastasis from non–small-cell lung carcinoma. The psychosomatic medicine service continued to follow the patient during the next 3 weeks. The patient was prescribed high-dosage steroids, and during his second week of hospitalization he received palliative intrathecal chemotherapy. The chemotherapy was stopped after several treatments because the patient developed altered mental status characterized by confusion and agitation. During his third week of hospitalization, the patient received several treatments of whole brain radiation. During this time the patient's neurological symptoms continued to progress, and he remained anxious, agitated, and confused, with worsening of symptoms at night. He told a psychiatry resident, "I feel like I'm going to die. I don't want to die." He developed a pulmonary embolism and a urinary tract infection.

The psychosomatic medicine service made medication recommendations regarding delirium and anxiety. Insertion of a feeding tube allowed for easier medication administration. The patient's agitation and disorientation were initially treated with olanzapine orally dissolving tablets, 2.5 mg twice daily and every 6 hours as needed for agitation (increased to 2.5 mg in the morning and 5 mg at night). Olanzapine was later switched to quetiapine (25 mg in the morning and 50 mg nightly) because of concerns about increased restlessness (possible akathisia) with olanzapine. Donepezil, which a number of case reports have shown effective for opiate-induced delirium, was also started at 5 mg nightly and increased to 10 mg after several days (Slatkin and Rhiner 2004; Slatkin et al. 2001).

The patient continued to have periodic confusion, but his agitation improved and lucid intervals were more common, allowing for supportive therapy. His female partner was at his bedside throughout his hospitalization, helping to reorient and soothe the patient. His last week of life was marked by several events that had special significance for the patient. By serendipitous coincidence, he received news that a multimedia production that he and his partner had recently completed had been accepted for a museum installation. The patient was proud of this achievement, which seemed especially meaningful given that it was a project that he and his partner had completed together. Additionally, the patient had several visitors, including a sister from whom he had been estranged, an old friend who had helped during his treatments for Hodgkin's disease in the distant past, and a rabbi. In a stance of acceptance of his imminent death and in increased closeness with significant others, he was preparing to go home with hospice care when he died.

◆ **Diagnosis: Axis I—Depressive Disorder Not Otherwise Specified, 311; Anxiety Disorder Not Otherwise Specified, 300.00; Delirium, 293.0**

The attending psychiatrist, third-year medical student, and psychiatry resident working with this patient found the case to be simultaneously difficult and rewarding in a number of ways. Each day was filled with new possibilities for treatment and, ultimately, failures of those treatments. The patient quickly moved from new cancer diagnosis to terminal stages of illness and developed new psychiatric symptoms throughout his stay. His poor prognosis became readily apparent even while various palliative treatments were being employed. The patient had little time to accept his diagnosis and to grieve his loss of self.

The complexities of medical pathology and treatment significantly affected the patient's mood and cognition and also made psychotropic medication selection and psychotherapy challenging. The finding of a second malignancy after treatment for Hodgkin's lymphoma is not unusual, because the relative risk of solid tumors, including lung cancer, in these patients is increased by more than twofold (Mauch 2008; van Leeuwen et al. 1994). Prognosis is generally poor in patients diagnosed with a second malignancy, particularly in patients with acute leukemia or lung cancer (Mauch 2008; Ng et al. 2002).

High rates of delirium are observed in patients during their last weeks of life (Minagawa et al. 1996). Alone, corticosteroids, cancer chemotherapy agents, and CNS disease can all result in myriad neuropsychiatric symptoms; in our patient, all of these factors were present. The patient's premorbid anxiety and mood disorders also likely added to his response to a new diagnosis. In choosing psychotropic medications for this patient, we had to consider his difficulty in swallowing without aspiration. Treatment was often limited to medications available in parenteral or orally dissolving forms. Dosage was also an uncertainty because the permeability of the patient's blood-brain barrier was almost certainly compromised by the CNS spread of his disease. Finally, drug–drug interactions were a significant concern because the patient was on a variety of chemotherapeutic agents and warfarin.

Although often complicated, the clinical work with this patient was in many ways inspiring for the psychosomatic medicine clinicians—we were able to observe a patient who appeared to successfully move through stages of grieving in an adaptive fashion within a very brief time period. The patient's evolving anxiety, mood, and cognitive symptoms were addressed both pharmacologically (with antidepressants, anxiolytics, atypical antipsychotics, and a cholinesterase inhibitor) and psychotherapeutically via supportive work with the patient and his partner. The psychosomatic medicine service encouraged the patient and his family toward a rapid fulfillment of various tasks—saying goodbye, establishing a legacy through his art, and achieving a spiritual peace. We were impressed and gratified to see the timely completion of the patient's generativity task via the museum project and joined in his celebrating this accomplishment.

Steinhauser et al. (2000) compared factors important to dying patients with those important to family members and healthcare practitioners. Factors that all three groups agreed were important involved pain and symptom management, preparation for the end of life, achieving a sense of completion, decisions about treatment preferences, and being treated as a "whole person." Factors valued by patients, and less so by physicians, included being mentally aware, having funeral arrangements planned, not being a burden, helping others, and coming to peace with God or another higher power.

Delirium Following Interleukin-2 Chemotherapy

The patient was a 57-year-old man with a history of renal cell carcinoma, status–post right nephrectomy, with metastatic disease to the lung. He also had a history of hypercholesterolemia, hypertension, and gastroesophageal reflux disease. He had no history of psychiatric illness. He was admitted to the medical center by the oncology service for a planned course of interleukin-2 for his metastatic disease. He was counseled on the numerous possible systemic side effects and began treatment.

He tolerated the first several doses well, but after the ninth dose, he developed cardiac dysfunction with reduced ejection fraction, renal failure, and fluid retention. While these systemic effects were being managed, he suddenly developed florid hyperactive delirium, characterized by motor agitation, pulling out of intravenous lines, confusion, altered sleep-wake cycle, yelling incoherently in his intensive care unit room, and disorientation. He claimed that he was in a hotel in his hometown, which was more than 100 miles from the medical center. He was also suspicious that the physicians and nurses were actively trying to harm him. His interleukin-2 was discontinued because of side effects.

Initial intensive-care treatment with opioids, haloperidol, and midazolam was ineffectual in controlling his agitated delirium; in fact, he became even more agitated after receiving these medications. He was also noted to have an increase in his QT_c interval from baseline; whether this was solely due to haloperidol could not be established. As his agitation and delirium progressed, he developed respiratory distress and was intubated and ventilated.

A psychosomatic medicine consultation was then requested. On examination, he was intubated and had variable level of consciousness. He could not respond reliably to simple questions with yes or no answers. He continued to be agitated and to have an altered sleep-wake cycle. Midazolam and haloperidol were discontinued, and he was treated with olanzapine 10 mg bid by nasogastric tube and 5 mg every 6 hours as needed for breakthrough agitation.

With further medical management, his cardiac function improved and his renal function returned to baseline levels. Over the next 4 days, his agitation resolved and he was extubated. He gradually recovered to his baseline mental status. His MMSE score at the time of medical discharge was 28. He was able to recall, in a patchy way, some of his delirium experiences, including a fear of being "assaulted" by hospital staff and having had florid visual hallucinations. His olanzapine was tapered and discontinued over a period of 10 days following his recovery of baseline mental status.

◆ **Diagnosis: Axis I—Delirium Due to Interleukin-2, 293.0**

Severe acute delirium has been associated with several chemotherapeutic agents, including interleukin-2 (Lerner et al. 1999). The neurotoxicity of these agents has not been associated with an exact mechanism. In addition to delirium, interleukin-2 has also been associated with mood changes, personality changes, concentration impairment, fatigue, and insomnia. This man had cardiac toxicity and renal failure in addition to delirium; it is unclear whether his delirium was secondary to these other systemic effects or primarily due to the "direct" neurotoxic effects of interleukin-2. Intervention with olanzapine, in concert with intensive care management of his cardiac and renal symptoms and discontinuation of interleukin-2, was correlated with steady improvement over a period of several days.

After recovery to normal baseline mental status, he was able to process some vivid memories of the disturbing delirium symptoms. Although he was still interested in pursuing alternative chemotherapy options for his metastatic cancer, he was concerned about developing another episode of delirium and was in discussions with the oncology service about his future chemotherapeutic options. Psychosomatic medicine psychiatrists working in oncology should be vigilant for acute delirium in the setting of new exposure to potentially neurotoxic chemotherapeutic agents.

The Two-Time Cancer Survivor With Residual Psychiatric Disorders

Cancer survivorship is a distinct identity. It may be more so for childhood cancer survivors. A compelling case was that of a two-time childhood cancer survivor who presented with what were, on thoughtful examination, quite plausible residual psychiatric symptoms. He responded well to an outpatient care model of psychotherapy and psychopharmacology.

> The patient was a 20-year-old white man who presented with difficulties learning in classroom settings and mild academic underachievement (symptoms of mild inattentive-type attention-deficit/hyperactivity disorder; ADHD), as well as shyness, social awkwardness, difficulty in confronting others, difficulty in initiating social relationships, and chronically mildly depressed mood. He had not previously been in psychiatric treatment.
>
> His medical history was quite remarkable. As a 6-year-old, he had had leukemia, from which he recovered after intensive and lengthy treatment with chemotherapy and bone marrow transplantation. As a result of his illness and treatment, he missed more than a year of school. When he reenrolled in school, his problems with inattention and social reticence conspired to limit his academic and social progress. Despite some early struggles, he was subsequently able to keep up with classmates, though with marginal performance and a year behind his age-matched peers.
>
> As a 13-year-old, he had another life-threatening illness. He developed osteosarcoma of the lower extremity. He needed extensive surgery, including reconstruction of leg bones to avoid an amputation. He also received additional intensive chemotherapy. Again, he lost a year of school. He recovered well. His residual condition was not significantly impaired; however, he had a noticeable limp and a loss of muscle mass of the affected lower extremity. His shyness and social reticence continued; these were additionally fueled by a sense of being conspicuously "different" as a result of his abnormal lower extremity.
>
> After his second cancer recovery, he was able to rejoin his classmates and eventually finished high school, albeit later than his similarly aged peers. He developed a keen interest in automotive

mechanics; when he presented for treatment, he had completed several months of a 2-year training program in automobile technology at a technical school, with a career goals of becoming an automobile service technician.

His psychiatric symptoms, although likely caused at least in part by the CNS toxicity of his chemotherapeutics, aggregated along the diagnoses of ADHD, inattentive type; dysthymic disorder; and avoidant personality disorder. Predictably, he was somewhat anxious about and slow to attach to the process of outpatient psychotherapy. He was, however, willing to take psychotropic medication for symptom improvement and to discuss his life experiences and goals for the future.

Despite his extraordinary tale of survival, he was not prone to complain over his medical history or to wallow in his past misery. Primarily, he now wanted to experience life as a normal 20-year-old man and did not want to identify himself as a "former cancer patient." He had a small circle of friends (many of whom shared his passion for Ford Mustangs), and he, to the degree he could, participated in "action" sports such as motocross and mountain biking. He possessed good insight; one of his primary motivations for treatment was to improve his mood and attention so as to be a better student in his technical school courses.

He was treated with bupropion to target his residual mood and attention symptoms. He tolerated a dosage of bupropion 150 mg sustained release twice a day without difficulty. He was able to notice improved attention and concentration; notably, he was now better able to learn his technical material from text sources. His mood also improved. From a stance of improved mood and attention, he was notably less shy and more eager to assert himself with peers, his girlfriend, and his family.

In psychotherapy sessions, he was able to put the cancer behind him and adopt a forward-looking and ultimately quite hopeful posture toward his career development, contemporary relationships, and a sense of a successful future. He was able to deal with his cancer history as having been an important part of his young life, but one that he did not want to be a defining identity object thereafter.

♦ **Diagnosis: Axis I—Attention-Deficit/Hyperactivity Disorder, Predominantly Inattentive Type, 314.00; Dysthymic Disorder, 300.4; Axis II—Avoidant Personality Disorder, 301.82**

When one deals with acutely ill cancer patients in the hospital, a clinical focus on adjustment to the devastating news of a new cancer diagnosis is often the first challenge. This may segue into acceptance of the illness and adoption of a "fighting stance" to accept treatment. The treatment phase may be helped considerably by the strong social support network characteristic of the cancer center model of treatment.

Less tangible, perhaps, are subtle but persistent neuropsychiatric symptoms following cancer treatment. Subtle cognitive, attention/concentration, and mood symptoms may follow chemotherapy or radiation treatment. In the relief and gratitude over cancer survival, such subtle residual symptoms may either not be appreciated or be quickly put into context as minor impairments. In this man's case, his attention and mood symptoms were likely at least partially referable to residual side effects of cancer interventions.

His avoidant personality disorder was likely at least in part a consequence of the prolonged separation from normal peer relationships at critical periods of psychological development at latency and adolescence; a synergy among ADHD, dysthymic disorder, and avoidant personality disorder is likely as well. The clinical approach of examining his various psychiatric symptoms in light of his medical history allowed for a comprehensive therapeutic approach. In the end, he was able to be the more socially functional 20-year-old he wished to be; his cancer survivorship was then less an object of primary identity and more a part of his past, not of his present and future.

The Struggles of the Survivor of a Cancer Victim: Substance Abuse, Boundary Issues, and Bereavement

A 64-year-old woman whose husband of 39 years had died 7 months earlier was referred to psychiatry when she disclosed she had been taking two sedatives without a formal recommendation. Her late husband was an orthopedic surgeon 2 years her junior who had been in excellent health until the incidental discovery of pancreatic cancer 4 months before his death. The patient said they had been "inseparable" since they first met. She was a nurse when they married but later earned a master's degree in business administration and had been his office manager for 22 years.

The patient described (since her husband's illness and death) persistent early-cycle insomnia, anhedonia, guilt over her decision to honor her husband's request for do-not-resuscitate status, and inertia draped with restless anxiety. She acknowledged weight loss, difficulty sustaining sufficient focus to read more than brief news items, and crying jags. Although she denied suicidal ideation, citing her religious faith, she added she did not see a future for herself.

The patient's insomnia had yielded to zolpidem, and her anxiety was eased by alprazolam. Although she had begun each at more moderate dosages, at the time of the evaluation she was taking zolpidem 20 mg each evening and alprazolam 2 mg four times daily. She had obtained the prescriptions from several different physician friends. Although she questioned her identity and purpose now that her husband was gone, she attended frequent social gatherings and parties, steadfastly refusing to speak about her grief with friends because "You must keep up your image!" The patient indignantly insisted she would not see a psychiatrist again, reasoning that her husband's colleagues understood her loss much more clearly and were therefore in a better position to prescribe anxiolytics and sleep aids.

♦ **Diagnosis: Axis I—Adjustment Disorder With Depressed Mood, 309.0, Versus Bereavement, V62.82; Rule Out Sedative, Hypnotic, or Anxiolytic Abuse, 305.40**

Depressed mood and associated symptoms in reaction to the death of a loved one are common. The duration and expression of grief vary widely and do not typically respect arbitrary time limits. It is not unusual for a survivor to encounter at least fleeting guilt related to some action or omission surrounding the death. Nor is it uncommon to have thoughts of death that center on a wish to join the deceased. However, a despondent preoccupation with worthlessness that impairs daily function on a prolonged basis is an uncharacteristic development. Similarly, hallucinations that go beyond seeing or hearing the departed loved one are unusual. Other clues that the survivor may be progressing to a complicated bereavement or major depressive episode include an apprehensive and intensive avoidance of reminders of the loss. The patient may perseverate on themes of disbelief or mournful yearning for the loved one that cannot be turned aside with other activities. The survivor may increasingly personalize feelings of worthlessness that extend well beyond the loss of the role she served in the prior relationship.

Although this patient endorsed multiple neurovegetative signs and symptoms in concert with her depressed mood, her range of social activities suggested her bereavement had not become a millstone of depression around her neck. Yet it had served to introduce her to the escapism provided by alprazolam and zolpidem to the point that she used multiple physician friends and various pharmacies to maintain a supply that supported her escalating usage. Part of the psychiatry consultant's challenge was to sufficiently understand and respect the magnitude of the loss so as to earn the privilege of speaking candidly about the mounting risks the patient was incurring. A useful question was, "What would your husband want you to do?" This gave the patient an opportunity to consider her situation from the vantage point of someone whose perspective she valued and trusted. She was less threatened by the imagined counsel of her deceased husband than by the words of the consultant present in her room.

References

Appelbaum PS, Grisso T: Assessing patients' capacities to consent to treatment. N Engl J Med 319:1635–1638, 1988

Balch CM, Buzaid AC, Soong S-J, et al: Final version of the American Joint Committee on Cancer staging system for cutaneous melanoma. J Clin Oncol 19:3635–3648, 2001

Brock DW: Voluntary active euthanasia. Hastings Cent Rep 22:10–22, 1992

Cassem E: Depressive disorders in the medically ill: an overview. Psychosomatics 36:S2–S10, 1995

Creasman WT, Odicino F, Maisonneuve P, et al: Carcinoma of the corpus uteri: FIGO annual report. Int J Gynaecol Obstet 83:79, 2003

Elkin TD, Phipps S, Mulhern RK, et al: Psychological functioning of adolescent and young adult survivors of pediatric malignancy. Med Pediatr Oncol 29:582–588, 1997

Folstein MF, Folstein SE, McHugh PR: "Mini-Mental State": a practical method for grading the cognitive state of patients for the clinician. J Psychiatr Res 12:189–198, 1975

Kleespies PL, Hughes DH, Gallacher FP: Suicide in the medically and terminally ill: psychological and ethical considerations. J Clin Psychol 56:1153–1171, 2000

Kübler-Ross E: On Death and Dying. New York, Routledge, 1973

Langeveld NE, Stam H, Grootenhuis MA, et al: Quality of life in young adult survivors of childhood cancer. Support Care Cancer 10:579–600, 2002

Lansky SB, List MA, Ritter-Sterr C: Psychosocial consequences of cure. Cancer 58:529–533, 1986

Lerner DM, Stoudemire A, Rosenstein DL: Neuropsychiatric toxicity associated with cytokine therapies. Psychosomatics 40:428–435, 1999

Mauch PM: Second malignancies after treatment of Hodgkin lymphoma. January 31, 2008. Available at http://www.uptodate.com/patients/content/topic.do?topicKey=lymphoma/8761. Accessed April 2, 2008.

Minagawa H, Uchitomi Y, Yamawaki S, et al: Psychiatric morbidity in terminally ill cancer patients: a prospective study. Cancer 78:1131–1137, 1996

Ng AK, Bernardo MV, Weller E, et al: Second malignancies after Hodgkin's disease treated with radiation therapy with or without chemotherapy: long-term risks and risk factors. Blood 100:1989, 2002

Slatkin N, Rhiner M: Treatment of opiate-induced delirium with acetylcholinesterase inhibitors: a case report. J Pain Symptom Manage 27:268–273, 2004

Slatkin NE, Rhiner M, Bolton TM: Donepezil in the treatment of opioid-induced sedation: a report of six cases. J Pain Symptom Manage 21:425–438, 2001

Steinhauser KE, Christakis NA, Clipp EC, et al: Factors considered important at the end of life by patients, family, physicians and other care providers. JAMA 284:2476–2482, 2000

Sullivan MD, Youngner SJ: Depression, competence, and the right to refuse lifesaving medical treatment. Am J Psychiatry 151:971–978, 1994

van Leeuwen FE, Klokman WJ, Hagenbeek A, et al: Second cancer risk following Hodgkin's disease: a 20-year follow-up study. J Clin Oncol 12:312, 1994

Wadzinski J, Franks R, Roane D, et al: Valproate-associated hyperammonemic encephalopathy. J Am Board Fam Med 20:499–502, 2007

Zeltzer LK, Chen E, Weiss R, et al: Comparison of psychologic outcome in adult survivors of childhood acute lymphoblastic leukemia versus sibling controls: a cooperative Children's Cancer Group and National Institutes of Health study. J Clin Oncol 15:547–556, 1997

RHEUMATOLOGY

Rheumatological illnesses are an obvious area for psychosomatic medicine interest. These illnesses are generally of long duration, cause significant functional impairment, and are associated with notably decreased quality of life and physical pain. In addition, comorbid psychiatric illnesses (notably mood disorders) are common in these patients. Beyond the psychiatric suffering associated with the underlying illnesses, the psychiatric side effects of systemic treatments (illustrated by the use of corticosteroids) are notable as well. Indeed, the psychiatrist will sometimes be asked to manage the medication-induced psychiatric side effects of these medications as a first encounter with a rheumatological patient. Finally, rheumatological illnesses may occasionally be the cause of mental status changes and thus are in the differential diagnosis of cases of cognitive impairment.

Systemic Lupus Erythematosus, Corticosteroids, and Mood Disorder

A 50-year-old female with a history of systemic lupus erythematosus, diabetes mellitus, chronic lymphedema, steroid-induced osteoporosis, and Raynaud's phenomenon was admitted to hospital with debilitating dyspnea and fatigue. The increase in these symptoms over the previous 2 weeks had led to a brisk escalation in her usual prednisone dose (from 20 mg to 60 mg daily) and was further supplemented with intravenous methylprednisolone.

Prior to her presentation to hospital, the patient complained of feeling nervous and unable to sit still. She described racing thoughts and harried feelings of hopelessness, prompting her to ask, "Am I losing my mind? Is this what happens when you go over the edge?" Her husband added that she had been uncharacteristically forgetful.

Despite fatigue, she was unable to sleep. Tearful without provocation, the patient said she was exhausted and felt she had "sand in my eyes." Her family physician was concerned that she may have been developing depression and initiated escitalopram. The patient denied a personal or family history of depression.

On examination, the patient was cushingoid in appearance but alert and fully oriented. She was restless in both demeanor and kinetics. Her speech alternated between brief bursts of a few sentences as she scurried through a particular thought and times of pensive, weary silence. Her thought processes were not uniformly linear. There was no evidence of first-rank Schneiderian symptoms. She described her mood as "uncomfortable" and appeared dysphoric as tears returned throughout the interview. She denied active suicidal ideation or intent but admitted she had thought it would be a relief if she could fall asleep at night and not waken. She scored 27 on the Mini-Mental State Examination (MMSE; Folstein et al. 1975), losing one point each on spelling backwards, the three-step command, and 5-minute recall.

In the hospital, the patient received lorazepam 1 mg every 4 hours over the first 2 days. The rheumatology service rapidly decreased her prednisone, and the patient noted dramatic improvement each day that the dosage was dropped. By the third hospital day, she was able to sleep throughout the night and was enormously relieved to discover this made an exceptional difference in her outlook and sense of well-being.

♦ **Diagnosis: Axis I—Mood Disorder Not Otherwise Specified, 296.90**

Steroids are known to precipitate a wide spectrum of psychiatric symptoms, ranging from acute dysphoria to euphoria with accompanying emotional lability that may result in weeping or giggling. Restlessness and agitation associated with increased distractibility and unfocused activity are commonplace. Insomnia and fragmented sleep often further exacerbate an already strained mental equilibrium. Because these patients are often contending with serious and chronic medical illnesses that involve multiple other medications and metabolic perturbations, frank psychosis is sometimes the presenting dilemma.

Benzodiazepines, antipsychotics, and mood stabilizers have all been deployed to good effect to treat corticosteroid-associated mood disturbances. In some situations when forthcoming corticosteroid use can be predicted and scheduled—for example, particular chemo-therapy protocols—it may be helpful to initiate prophylaxis with a mood stabilizer or other psychotropic agent several days in advance.

Takayasu's Arteritis, Rheumatoid Arthritis, Depression, and Psychosis

A 48-year-old woman presented unaccompanied to her rheumatol-ogist's office with uncharacteristic affect and peculiar speech. The rheumatologist made a quick phone call, and the patient was es-corted to the waiting room of a nearby psychiatrist. When her name was called, she stood slowly and walked with a studied gait as if fol-lowing an unseen line across the floor. Safely in the psychiatrist's of-fice, she sat down gingerly and perched awkwardly on the forward edge of the chair. Her demeanor was distracted and perplexed. After scanning the walls briefly, she offered a hesitant, slowly extracted history of deepening dysphoria with associated anxiety and visual hallucinations. She offered virtually no eye contact for the first 45 minutes of the interview and often simply stared off into space. She spoke in choppy fragments of phrases with long pauses between words. At times she repeated a short phrase several times with the raspy, repetitive rhythm of a broken record player before she would skip to an alternate "groove" and answer a question appropriately. She chewed on her thumb, and her legs were restless. Her voice had a simple, child-like quality. Her solemn facial expressions seemed to reflect an internal fight to untangle her thought processes.

She initially said that she had come because of "Kinda repeating thoughts…kinda to even out my mood…because I'm anxious…and if my head slowed down I could get a break." With enormous effort, she went on to detail that she had experienced an increasingly de-pressed mood for several weeks, accompanied by mild early morn-ing awakening, less initiative and motivation than she normally enjoyed, exhaustion, colliding and difficult-to-organize thoughts, and a "wish that I could be mentally clean and erase all of my thoughts." The patient firmly denied suicidal ideation or intent. She acknowledged wishing at times that she could have an extended sleep to recuperate from her sense of exhaustion. She also confessed that her thoughts were "dirty" and that she wished all her thoughts could be erased but reiterated that she did not think dying would be necessary to "erase the thoughts." She repeated several times that she felt dirty, as though disclosing this somehow set the stage for the "washing and erasing" that she slowly insisted was necessary. De-spite long pauses and apparent attempts to summon words to expand on these comments, she lapsed into silence over and again. Eventually, she blurted out that the dirty thoughts included "Seeing something that happened to you…something from college…something from a kid…a whole bunch of stuff," but she went on to deny ever experiencing any abuse or other trauma. She retreated to silence once again, broken only to say these thoughts were very private.

Later, she interrupted a review of past medical history to volunteer that her thoughts were "really not thoughts…they are little short movies…kinda make me sick…nauseated sick." She explained that these "little short movies" were not silent, but they contained no talking, either. Rather, she said she was able to hear "him…no talking…just bad noises." She denied any command hallucinations. The patient said similar episodes had occurred several times in the past and she had been hospitalized in another state, although the last incident had been 4 years ago. She recalled taking fluoxetine (Prozac) for several years with some benefit with respect to mood, but she had then become convinced it was associated with weight gain and discontinued it. She also remembered taking sertraline (Zoloft) 1 year earlier, but in spite of a beneficial effect on her mood she had again become concerned that it was associated with weight gain and thus discontinued it. She recognized olanzapine (Zyprexa), quetiapine (Seroquel), and risperidone (Risperdal) as three agents that had been helpful with the "little short movies" but that were also associated with weight gain, prompting her to discontinue them.

The patient scored 28 on the MMSE, missing only the date and one item on 5-minute recall. She managed serial 7s accurately but literally required 3 minutes of earnest concentration to do so. It took almost 2 minutes for her to write the sentence, "I live in Arcola, Illinois."

The patient hesitated before revealing that during college in her early 20s she had developed bulimia nervosa and remembered that her maximum weight at the time was between 140 and 150 pounds. A couple of years after earning her bachelor's degree, she became severely anorectic and her weight dropped to between 70 and 80 pounds before a prolonged hospitalization helped her recover metabolic equilibrium. She observed that her weight was now 125 pounds and, although comfortable with this weight, was emphatic that she did not wish to gain so much as "one pound more." She said she no longer restricted or purged in any fashion and had not had any behaviors indicative of an active eating disorder for nearly 4 years.

The patient's presentation to a rheumatologist was no accident. Diagnosed with juvenile rheumatoid arthritis, she later developed Takayasu's arteritis and had a 22-year history of recurring bouts that had required episodic high-dose steroids and other potent immuno-suppressants. She also had a history of hypertension and vascular headaches but no previous psychiatric diagnoses apart from the eating disorder mentioned earlier. At the time of her referral to psychiatry, she was taking aspirin 325 mg daily; mycophenolate 1,000 mg twice daily; risedronate 35 mg once weekly; and topiramate 200 mg twice daily. Apart from a single cup of caffeinated coffee per day, she avoided stimulants of any kind. She had never smoked and only drank wine at Christmas.

The patient was born and raised in the rural Midwest as the second of three children in an intact farm family, which she recalled in favorable terms. She denied any abuse whatsoever during childhood or adolescence and recalled that she had had none of her symptoms of eating disorder until she entered college. She had taught third grade for a year before choosing to marry and remain at home. She had two children and described a good relationship with her husband. She was unaware of any history of psychiatric illness in her extended family.

Over the years, the patient had presented her physicians in rheumatology, neurology, and vascular surgery with multiple challenges. When she was 26 years old, she developed upper extremity claudication and recurring visual scotomata and tunnel vision. After evaluation, she underwent an aortobilateral carotid artery bypass graft. A year later, symptoms of posterior circulation insufficiency prompted a saphenous vein graft from the aortic arch to the right vertebral artery. Subsequent reocclusions (at 1 week and 4 years later) required extensive revisions of these bypasses. Her abdominal aorta and lower extremity vasculature were largely unaffected, but she later developed a complete occlusion of the right vertebral artery, and the ascending aorta stretched to 4.8 cm in diameter. Her multiple grafts were strained by pseudoaneurysms bulging exteriorly and ulcerations noted internally.

In addition to her juvenile rheumatoid arthritis and Takayasu's arteritis, the patient had developed a seizure disorder that bedeviled her and her physicians because of its often varying presentations. She had only rare generalized motor symptoms. More commonly, her symptoms were consistent with complex partial seizures. Infrequently, her symptoms were more unusual; for example, she once went through a car wash in a convertible but did not remember to raise the top before commencing the wash. She later described having felt as if she were in a dissociated state, being vaguely aware that she ought to put up the top but feeling removed from caring sufficiently to take the initiative to do so. Her family described times when she "stared into space," and the patient struggled to describe these beyond saying she felt "different and odd." Over the years, she had had some electroencephalograms that showed epileptogenic activity, others that were normal, and some that revealed grade I dysrhythmias with generalized slowing.

High-dose steroids, cyclophosphamide, methotrexate, infliximab, and mycophenolate had all been used at various times alongside a variety of nonsteroidal anti-inflammatory and antiepileptic drugs. She had no family psychiatric history, and most, but not every, episode of depression had been temporally associated with a flare in either joint symptoms (e.g., morning stiffness, swollen knuckles, and pain) or laboratory markers of increased arterial inflammation (e.g., elevations in erythrocyte sedimentation rate and/or C-reactive protein). Her clinical exacerbations had typically been precipitous and not immediately reversed. For this reason, when depression (with or without accompanying psychotic symptoms) occurred alongside her rheumatological illness, it was treated with psychotropic medication; the patient had never been treated solely with steroids and immunosuppressants to assess the response of depression to these agents alone. Although not all records were available for review, the patient denied ever experiencing psychotic symptoms independent of either depression or symptoms of Takayasu's arteritis.

◆ **Diagnosis: Axis I—Depressive Disorder Not Otherwise Specified (With Psychotic Features), 311; Eating Disorder Not Otherwise Specified (in Remission), 307.50**

This patient illustrates the complex interplay of multiple factors: the psychosocial context of a chronic, debilitating illness that first intruded and disrupted her life as an active teenager; the subsequent emergence of Takayasu's arteritis, which led to an interminable list of complex vascular surgeries that repeatedly threatened her brain function and required sustained commitment to medications with their own adverse potentials; a polymorphic seizure disorder that not only defied predictability but also required medications that shaped her energy, initiative, and cognition; and a recurrent depressive illness that was often associated with psychosis.

Following hospitalization, yet another complicating element was discovered when further collateral history became available: there was reliable evidence that the patient had experienced serious and prolonged sexual abuse during her early childhood. Further history emerged piecemeal, because the patient's home was far removed from the medical center where she was ultimately hospitalized. One challenge her local physicians faced was whether her arteritis contributed to her depression or if the reverse was the more plausible sequence.

At first glance, the temporal sequence appeared to implicate a surge in joint and other rheumatological symptoms before dysphoria appeared. However, the patient's mycophenolate level was subtherapeutic on admission, and as her systemic symptoms improved, she revealed there were at least some occasions when she experienced progressive paranoia in concert with depression. These occasions prompted her to become suspicious that her immunosuppressants represented a life-threatening conspiracy, and she would begin to take them erratically. Thus it may have been that her depression, accompanied by increasing suspicion and fear, led to noncompliance and consequent flares in her rheumatoid arthritis and Takayasu's arteritis.

The patient responded to an increase in prednisone, titration of mycophenolate (CellCept) to achieve a therapeutic level, and initiation of aripiprazole and citalopram. Her paranoia receded gradually but completely, although her depression intensified briefly as she learned how ill she had been. With the resolution of her delusional conviction that the immunosuppressants represented a lethal plot against her, she no longer balked or refused these medications, and the laboratory markers of arteritis returned to normal levels.

Reference

Folstein MF, Folstein SE, McHugh PR: "Mini-Mental State": a practical method for grading the cognitive state of patients for the clinician. J Psychiatr Res 12:189–198, 1975

10

INFECTIOUS DISEASES

Some of the most challenging and interesting psychosomatic medicine cases are patients with infectious disease. Whether they are the main reason for hospitalization or they occur as a common complication of other medical and surgical illness, infectious diseases remain a major scourge of hospitalized patients. Infectious diseases may be associated with psychiatric illnesses in many contexts. Direct central nervous system (CNS) infection may cause the acute presentation of psychiatric symptoms; this can be especially striking when the psychiatric symptoms occur without motor or other neurological symptoms. Localized or systemic infections may lead to delirium, which requires its own evaluation and managements. Infectious diseases may be treated with pharmacological agents that are themselves associated with CNS (including psychiatric) side effects.

The HIV/AIDS epidemic beginning in the 1980s has been one of the major events in contemporary medicine and has spawned much research and progress in clinical care. The psychosomatic medical care of HIV/AIDS patients has grown accordingly, to where, in some academic institutions, there are psychosomatic medicine services focused primarily on the care of these patients. HIV/AIDS remains one of the more common causes of cognitive impairment in young patients. The infection of the CNS with HIV may be associated with mental status changes in advance of evidence of immunosuppression. HIV/AIDS patients have a high prevalence of mood disorders that may require individualized psychopharmacological approaches.

As HIV/AIDS has progressed to become more of a chronic disease in many cases, issues of medication and clinical compliance, adaptation and adjustment to a chronic illness, and other areas have become increasingly important. HIV/AIDS will likely remain an area of great interest to the psychosomatic medicine field for generations to come.

Malignant Catatonia and Viral Encephalitis

The patient, a 31-year-old white female laboratory-technician student, previously in good health, experienced the onset of a severe, pounding headache and presented to an outside emergency room. A head computed tomography (CT) scan was negative. She was sent home, but the headache persisted. Five days later, the patient's family noted that she had become confused and agitated, resisted attempts to be calmed, and appeared to be hallucinating. They brought her back to the emergency department, where she now demonstrated disorganized thoughts that were attributed to hydrocodone she had taken for the headache. She was again sent home, but 6 hours later, the family brought her back. The patient said she was "going to die in 30 minutes" and talked about the "different stages my brain is going through."

Vital signs (including temperature) were normal; physical examination was remarkable for agitation, nonsensical speech, delusions, and disorientation. She had no history of alcohol or illicit drug use. A lumbar puncture, repeat head CT, and urine and blood screenings were done, and the patient was transported to a referral hospital for admission to the psychiatry unit for treatment of acute psychosis.

On the psychiatry inpatient unit, the patient continued to be agitated, was oriented to person only, and had disorganized tangential speech. Collateral history revealed that earlier in the week she had been febrile and nauseated and had vomited. Two hours after her admission to the psychiatric unit, additional outside laboratory results became available. Blood and urine toxicology were unrevealing, but lumbar puncture showed her glucose to be 66 mg/dL, protein 127 mg/dL, red blood cells 0 per mm^3, and white blood cells 336 per mm^3 with 83% lymphocytes, 13% monocytes, and 4% other cells. An electroencephalogram showed moderately severe generalized slow wave abnormalities without focal or lateralizing features.

Assumed to have a working diagnosis of meningoencephalitis, the patient was transferred to the internal medicine floor and received intravenous acyclovir and prophylactic antimicrobials, including antituberculins. By the next day, she could not follow directions, did not communicate verbally, and became so severely combative that she required six staff members to physically restrain her. To control agitation, 13 mg of intravenous lorazepam was given in the first 36 hours, without sufficient benefit. She was transferred to the medical intensive care unit, where the medical team opted to sedate her with intravenous propofol, lorazepam, and midazolam. Esmolol was started for new-onset atrial fibrillation.

Over the next 2 days, attempts to taper either the propofol or benzodiazepines resulted in increased agitation. In addition, autonomic instability characterized by dramatic excursions in blood pressure and heart rate as well as tachypnea and a temperature of 38.2°C emerged. The patient displayed catatonic posturing, rigidity, staring, negativism, mutism, immobility/stupor, and episodes of excitement/impulsivity and combativeness. In an attempt to calm her, the patient was given a total of 1.5 mg of haloperidol intravenously, but she remained agitated. She was intubated the next day to protect her airway and was noted to have increased muscle tone, a slight tremor, and hyperreflexia of all limbs. Benzodiazepines were used for agitation control, with moderate efficacy.

Over the next 8 days, the patient continued to be alternately combative and stuporous. She was mute with persistent staring and displayed negativism, profound rigidity, posturing, and stereotypic behaviors. She was febrile to 39.2°C and markedly diaphoretic, with her heart rate ranging from 46 to 200 beats per minute and systolic blood pressures from 105 to 180 mm Hg. Over the next 3 days, she received five doses of haloperidol, 2.5 mg intravenously each, in addition to the propofol. Her temperature rose to 40.0°C within 24 hours of the last dose, she had repetitive chewing movements, and she experienced three episodes of asystole, each lasting 8–12 seconds.

Psychiatry was consulted to help with the patient's agitation. Malignant catatonia secondary to presumptive viral encephalitis was diagnosed. (Interestingly, no viral pathogen was ever isolated.) Neurology proposed a trial of morphine sulfate (to be administered 10 mg intravenously every 30 minutes for a total of three doses), but it resulted in little more than an abatement of rigors. Given the grave outcome of previous cases of untreated malignant catatonia and this patient's progressive downward course despite aggressive benzodiazepine treatment, the psychiatry team elected to proceed with emergent electroconvulsive therapy (ECT).

The patient received the first two bilateral ECT treatments in rapid succession. Within 4 hours, she showed mild improvement in hemodynamic stability; however, during the night she exhibited marked rigidity with decerebrate posturing. Emergent head CT was negative. The next day, the patient received her third ECT treatment and was more alert and less rigid by the following morning. On the third day, she received a fourth ECT treatment and thereaf-

ter appeared to follow some simple verbal commands. She was extubated that morning, but by evening, she had difficulty protecting
her airway and required reintubation.

The next day, a fifth ECT treatment was given, and she was later
treated for supraventricular tachycardia with Wolff-Parkinson-
White-like characteristics. Two days later, the patient was given a
sixth ECT treatment. She subsequently had good eye contact and
tracking, with very little residual rigidity, and twice had a hint of a
smile in response to humor. A seventh ECT treatment was given the
next day after some autonomic fluctuations were noted overnight.
An evolving methicillin-resistant *Staphylococcus aureus* pneumonia
delayed further ECT for 5 days. Despite this, she was alert and responsive, obeyed commands, spent several hours in a chair, tracked
well, and had more purposeful movements.

By the fifth day after her last ECT treatment, she was once again
more rigid, displayed definite waxy flexibility, and had decreased eye
contact, so an eighth ECT treatment was given. That night, she attempted to communicate with staff, followed complex commands including playing patty-cake, and waved to staff outside of the room.
Within 4 subsequent days, she had become agitated again, with slight
rigidity and posturing, and so was given a ninth ECT treatment. The
patient again showed improvement for 5 days, but on the sixth day,
she was again rigid, with repetitive motoric marching activity and periodic waxy flexibility; a tenth ECT treatment was then given. Thereafter, she had persistent, progressive improvement in all spheres. She
started eating and talking within 5 days of the last treatment and required only lorazepam to aid sleep and control restlessness.

Six weeks after her admission to the intensive care unit, she was
transferred to the physical medicine and rehabilitation unit for
14 days. After hospital discharge, she received outpatient speech and
physical rehabilitation therapies for 5 months. The lorazepam tapered and discontinued within 2 months. Cognitive testing after discharge revealed deficits in a number of areas. However, neurocognitive testing performed 5 months later showed considerable
improvement with "no strong evidence for clinically significant neurocognitive deficits." Her catatonia did not recur, and the patient
had no cause for further psychiatric contact in the ensuing 3 years.

◆ **Diagnosis: Axis I—Catatonic Disorder Due to a General
Medical Condition, 293.89; Psychotic Disorder Not
Otherwise Specified, 298.9; Delirium, 293.0**

This case is a striking example of how catatonia, with its syndro-
mal cluster of signs, can arise not only in the setting of psychoses or

mood disorders but also amid medical and neurological insults to the body and brain. Catatonia is considered malignant when the clinical picture includes hyperthermia and autonomic instability.

Although the patient was initially referred with what was believed to be a functional psychosis, cerebrospinal fluid abnormalities and the rapid decline in her medical status suggested a viral etiology. Progress notes from the medical floor and intensive care unit documented the presence of rigidity, posturing, staring, negativism, mutism, stupor/immobility, and combativeness in the first 3 days of hospitalization. Her subsequent progression to malignant catatonia, with the cardinal signs of autonomic instability (including erratic excursions in blood pressure, heart rate, and respirations) and elevated temperature, clearly preceded her initial exposure to antipsychotics. The observation of increased rigidity after haloperidol administration, however, suggests that the intravenous haloperidol used for behavioral control may have exacerbated the progression of her malignant catatonia. This further illustrates the potential danger of treating progressive catatonia with antipsychotics.

The clinical signs of catatonia in medical patients without psychiatric illness, in psychiatric patients without antipsychotic exposure, and in patients exposed to antipsychotics are nearly indistinguishable. It is probable that despite different origins, these syndromes merge because they share a final common pathway of altered neurophysiology.

In this patient's case, a distinct cause for her malignant catatonia was never identified and therefore could not be specifically treated. However, her case demonstrates that all dopamine antagonists (regardless of the etiology of the catatonic features) must be eliminated from the treatment of this condition. Clinical experience has shown benzodiazepines to be beneficial in such cases. This patient's sustained exposure to high-dosage benzodiazepines may have been what kept her alive until psychiatry was consulted and ECT initiated. Numerous sources show ECT to be particularly helpful for malignant catatonia, with rapid stabilization and recovery in the majority of the patients treated. In this patient's case, her symptoms remitted steadily with continued ECT treatments, the frequency of which was guided by the severity of continuing motor signs of catatonia. The last of these signs eventually yielded to low-dosage lorazepam.

Malignant catatonia likely represents the final common pathway of severely altered neurobiology (with prominent contributions from dopaminergic and γ-aminobutyric acid [GABA]-ergic pathways) that can occur in either medical or psychiatric illness, with and without the potentially aggravating factor of antipsychotics or other dopa-active medications.

This patient's case serves as a signal reminder that catatonia may occur in medical/surgical units and that consultation psychiatrists are uniquely equipped to contribute to its management. Aggressive utilization of ECT may be lifesaving for patients with catatonia despite the absence of "psychiatric history" or other conventional indications for ECT. Benzodiazepines have an important adjunctive role, as might other dopa-active or muscle-relaxant drugs.

Improved and prompt recognition of malignant catatonia in the medical setting will not only strengthen the care of these patients but may also enable advances in the study, understanding, and treatment of catatonia occurring in the context of psychiatric illness and pharmacological interventions.

Neurocysticercosis With Mood and Psychotic Symptoms

The patient was a 50-year-old Hispanic female with a 20-year history of hydrocephalus. She had had a ventriculo-peritoneal shunt placed early in her illness. She had a long history of depression with neurovegetative signs and recently had been treated with venlafaxine extended release 150 mg every morning. A new magnetic resonance imaging (MRI) scan revealed a temporal lobe cystic mass with increased midline shift. A ventriculostomy, temporal cyst aspiration, and biopsy of temporal lobe lesions were done shortly before psychosomatic medicine clinical evaluation. After examination of the pathological specimen and an infectious disease consultation, neurocysticercosis was diagnosed. She was then treated with rifampin, vancomycin, and albendazole.

Shortly after the neurosurgical procedure, she began to experience new psychotic symptoms. She had visual hallucinations of seeing a "dead dog" in her hospital room and auditory hallucinations of hearing voices of her children speaking to her. She also abruptly got up from her hospital bed and got dressed, insisting that she had to "get to work." Upon psychosomatic medicine evaluation, she displayed anxiously tearful affect and had a Mini-Mental State Examination (MMSE; Folstein et al. 1975) score of 26. She was treated with low-dosage risperidone 0.5 mg twice a day, and her venlafaxine was continued. Over the next several days, her mood improved, she no longer reported perceptual disturbances, and she did not exhibit any more confusion. Her MMSE score improved to 30.

◆ **Diagnosis: Axis I—Major Depressive Disorder, Recurrent, Severe Without Psychotic Features, 296.33; Psychotic Disorder Not Otherwise Specified, 298.9**

Neurocysticercosis results from neural tissue infection with larval *Taenia solium*. Neuropsychiatric symptoms associated with this condition include increased intracranial pressure, hydrocephalus, seizures, cognitive impairment, psychosis, and mood disturbances. Psychiatric symptoms may be the presenting physical symptom in some patients. Progression of the systemic disease has been associated with progression of neuropsychiatric symptoms; paradoxically, the institution of antiparasitic drugs, associated with increased CNS inflammation, may also lead to increased neuropsychiatric symptoms.

This woman had had hydrocephalus for 20 years, including early ventriculo-peritoneal shunting for increased intracranial pressure. Despite this recognition of hydrocephalus and neurosurgical intervention, she had not been formally diagnosed with neurocysticercosis. Her onset of depression was during the time of her onset of hydrocephalus; in retrospect, it is a plausible formulation that her longstanding depression was a neuropsychiatric manifestation of neurocysticercosis.

Twenty years later, when she presented with cognitive symptoms of confusion and poor concentration, associated with nausea and headache, full evaluation led to repeated neurosurgical intervention and an eventual tissue diagnosis of recurrent neurocysticercosis. However, for the period of her illness, she did not appear to have been psychotic until treatment for her infection was finally initiated.

Although it is difficult to prove causally, this sequence of clinical events is consistent with some of the literature to connect the acute psychosis to the effects of antimicrobial therapy. Empirical treatment with risperidone was associated with significant symptomatic improvement.

Psychosomatic medicine physicians encountering patients with this infectious disease are reminded of the association of neurocysticercosis with a wide range of neuropsychiatric symptoms. Full psychiatric evaluation, cognitive assessment, and neuroimaging are essential parts of comprehensive care. Empirical use of psychopharmacological agents for the specific psychiatric symptoms is encouraged, and monitoring for change in severity and/or type of psychiatric symptoms is necessary as the disease progresses and/or responds to intervention.

Isoniazid and Psychosis

Case 1

The patient was a 60-year-old Filipino woman who had recently moved to the United States. Although conversant in English, she was a primary Tagalog speaker. She was admitted to the medical center for abdominal pain and bowel obstruction; she subsequently had an uncomplicated partial small bowel resection. She had been started on isoniazid for a positive tuberculosis test 3 weeks earlier.

She had a psychosomatic medicine consultation ordered for "odd behavior and paranoia." She had reported to nursing staff that there was "something strange" in her bathroom. In addition, she was hallucinating images in her hospital room of people she had known in the Philippines. Because of these images, she was frightened to stay in her hospital room and would sit for hours at the nurses' station. She also claimed that threatening voices were "coming from the walls." She made several telephone calls to her family requesting that they "rescue" her from the medical center. She had no history of psychiatric illness.

Upon examination, she claimed that "strange men" were sleeping in her hospital bed and threatening her. She was neither suicidal nor homicidal. Her MMSE score was 19. She was notably distractible but not disorganized. Level of consciousness was full.

Because of the possible relationship between isoniazid and psychotic symptoms, the patient's isoniazid was discontinued. She was also treated with low-dosage risperidone, 1 mg twice a day. Pyridoxine supplementation was also added. Within 2 days, her hallucinations and delusions had resolved, and her cognitive status had returned to normal, with a follow-up MMSE score of 30. Upon her recovery, risperidone was weaned and discontinued after 3 weeks and without recurrence of psychotic symptoms.

◆ **Diagnosis: Axis I—Psychotic Disorder Not Otherwise Specified, 298.9**

Case 2

The second patient was a 25-year-old Filipino male who developed a positive purified protein derivative test; he had no history of active tuberculosis. He was started on prophylactic isoniazid 300 mg every morning. Four months later, he developed irritably dysphoric mood, poor concentration, paranoid ideation (e.g., a new concern, unsubstantiated, that his wife's friend had become a "communist"), and resultant social-occupational difficulties. He denied other psychiatric history or symptoms. When evaluated, he claimed that the interviewer had made threatening gestures toward him and expressed concerns that the interviewer was trying to "hypnotize and control" him.

At this point, isoniazid was discontinued. He was not treated with antipsychotic medications. Over the next 2 weeks, his psychotic symptoms resolved completely; on subsequent evaluation, he had no paranoid ideations, euthymic and nonlabile affect, normal attention and concentration, and an MMSE score of 30. Physical examination, MRI scans, electroencephalograms, and formal psychological testing were all normal. He looked back on his brief period of psychotic symptoms with some perplexity but was able to clearly identify that the paranoid ideations were, in retrospect, quite foreign to his habitual percepts and understanding and that he felt he had returned to his normal baseline after isoniazid was discontinued.

◆ **Diagnosis: Axis I—Psychotic Disorder Not Otherwise Specified, 298.9**

These cases illustrate the connection between an antitubercular medication (isoniazid) and medication-induced psychotic symptoms. These patients were not delirious: they maintained normal level of consciousness, did not exhibit disturbances of the circadian rhythm, and did not have motor agitation. Once isoniazid was discontinued and low-dosage risperidone was started in the first case, the patient's psychotic symptoms promptly improved and she was able to perform much better on the cognitive examination. The second patient did not require antipsychotic medication, because the psychosis cleared promptly with discontinuation of isoniazid. Psychosomatic medicine psychiatrists treating patients exposed to antitubercular medications should consider this relationship, encourage their infectious diseases colleagues to consider alternative antituberculars in patients experiencing psychosis with isoniazid, and monitor cognitive and psychotic symptoms closely as patients are taken off of isoniazid.

HIV/AIDS, Delirium, and Depression

Cases of HIV are associated with varying degrees of complex and often overlapping psychiatric illnesses. A clinical approach to these patients often requires the creative use of psychopharmacology and psychotherapeutic approaches.

> A 35-year-old man with HIV/AIDS, hepatitis B infection, and hypothyroidism presented to a community hospital with a small bowel obstruction. A peritoneal abscess drained during exploratory laparotomy was later found to contain mycobacterium tuberculosis. He was quickly transferred to a university medical center for treatment of tuberculous peritonitis. The patient's course was complicated by the development of several enterocutaneous fistulae, *Clostridium difficile* colitis, and poor nutritional status. He received parenteral nutrition, and medications were delivered primarily by cutaneous patch and intravenously. His medications included a scopolamine patch, fentanyl patch, hydromorphone patient-controlled intravenous analgesia, zolpidem, morphine, metoclopramide, famotidine, promethazine, levoxyl, several antibiotics, and pyridoxine.
>
> Five weeks into his hospitalization, and 6 days after a repeat exploratory laparotomy, the patient appeared increasingly anxious and confused. The primary surgery team was concerned about this change in mental status and requested a psychosomatic medicine consult. On initial evaluation, the patient complained of increased nervousness and insomnia since his most recent surgery. The patient's mother added that he had been hallucinating and appearing intermittently confused for several days.
>
> The patient had a history of major depression, without mania or psychosis, that had been treated intermittently for the previous 10 years. He had no prior history of anxiety disorder. His prior psychotropic medications included fluoxetine, sertraline, and duloxetine, none of which he thought were particularly helpful and all of which had been discontinued. He admitted to a history of methamphetamine dependence, which had been in complete remission for 4½ years. He had contracted HIV 11 years earlier via unprotected sex with men and had been diagnosed for the past 1½ years with AIDS.
>
> On examination, the patient was pleasant but disheveled and inattentive, with frequent thought derailment and apparent response to internal stimuli. He was notably restless and had a coarse tremor

and frequent myoclonic jerks. His initial MMSE score was 26. The psychosomatic medicine team diagnosed delirium, major depression by history, and anxiety disorder not otherwise specified and recommended a revision of the patient's medications, including discontinuation of the scopolamine patch and minimization of short-acting opiates, benzodiazepines, and zolpidem. Various studies were recommended, including head CT scan, serum ammonia, vitamin B_{12} level, folate, rapid plasma reagin, and surveillance for additional sources of infection. The team also recommended initiating treatment with olanzapine orally dissolving tablet 2.5 mg twice a day and 2.5 mg every 6 hours as needed for agitation.

In the week after the initial psychosomatic medicine evaluation, the patient experienced a worsening of confusion and hallucinations; his MMSE score declined to 21. He had continued to receive treatment with patient-controlled hydromorphone, but the scopolamine patch and zolpidem were discontinued. Family members remarked that the patient's hallucinations clearly increased about 1 hour after each hydromorphone dose but that this medication was the only one that adequately controlled his pain. Serum ammonia was elevated at 50 μmol/L, thyroid-stimulating hormone was mildly elevated at 6.77 mU/L with a normal free T4; B_{12}, folate, head CT scan, and rapid plasma reagin were normal /nonreactive. The patient had continued to have fevers and was diagnosed with recurrent *Clostridium difficile* colitis and right-sided pneumonia, which were treated with additional antibiotics. He was also found to have a new perforation in his small intestine and another enterocutaneous fistula. His olanzapine was increased gradually to an eventual dosage of 5 mg every morning and 7.5 mg at bedtime for persistent delirium. He remained on this regimen for several days with no appreciable improvement in orientation or lessening of agitation.

Ten days after initial psychiatric evaluation, the psychosomatic medicine team recommended the initiation of an acetylcholinesterase inhibitor, donepezil, to treat opiate-induced confusion. Case reports of patients with similar characteristics suggested that this medication might be useful (Slatkin and Rhiner 2004; Slatkin et al. 2001). Donepezil, in orally dissolving form (chosen because of the patient's poor tolerance of oral medications and unreliable gastrointestinal absorption), was started at 5 mg at bedtime. Within 4 days of treatment, the patient's MMSE score had returned to 28, and 2 days later it was 30. His hallucinations had resolved despite continuation of hydromorphone.

After the patient's delirium had cleared, he was able to communicate articulately the extent of his depression. Mirtazapine 15 mg at bedtime, also in orally dissolving form, was prescribed for insomnia and depression. This was titrated up to 30 mg at bedtime several weeks after initiation. The patient's anxiety had resolved with the resolution of the delirium. Olanzapine was tapered and discontinued. Although the patient had a normal head CT scan, a head MRI performed several weeks later showed "flair hyperintensity in the periventricular white matter, especially right frontal and splenium of corpus callosum, which may be secondary to HIV encephalitis or progressive multifocal leukoencephalopathy (PML)." The patient was restarted on combined antiretroviral therapy (CART) before discharge from the hospital. His total length of stay was 5 months.

◆ **Diagnosis: Axis I—Delirium, 293.0; Major Depressive Disorder, Recurrent, Moderate, 296.32; Anxiety Disorder Not Otherwise Specified, 300.00; Amphetamine Dependence, 304.40**

This case demonstrates the complex interplay of infectious disease, pharmacology, and psychopathology that are often involved in the care of patients with HIV/AIDS. Studies have shown increased rates of serious mental illness, including schizophrenia, major affective disorders (Walkup et al. 1999), and personality disorders, in various HIV-positive populations (Klinkenberg and Sacks 2004; Perkins et al. 1993) as well as increased rates of lifetime diagnosis of any drug or alcohol use disorder compared with the general population (Klinkenberg and Sacks 2004).

Persons living with HIV and AIDS may also experience a number of neuropsychiatric symptoms, including deficits in attention, concentration, and motor function, which have been found to worsen with the progression of disease (Reger et al. 2002). HIV enters the CNS soon after infection, and infection may result in acute meningitis, vacuolar myelopathy, peripheral neuropathy, and myopathy (Berger and Brew 2005; Simpson 1998). Many of the antiretroviral agents used to treat HIV infection are associated with neuropsychiatric symptoms and may also interact with psychotropic medications. Other infections associated with AIDS include several that directly affect the CNS and can lead to neuropsychiatric symptoms, such as toxoplasmosis, cytomegalovirus, PML, cryptococcal meningitis, and neurosyphilis (Simpson 1998); the antimicrobials used to treat these opportunistic infections can also lead to such symptoms. Additionally, the psychological stress of having a disease that is often debilitating and fatal can cause its own difficulties with adjustment and hopelessness. Patients with AIDS may be especially sensitive to the CNS effects of medications and the development of delirium due to preexisting HIV-related CNS pathology. Delirium in patients with HIV/AIDS has been associated with increased mortality, longer hospital stay, and greater dependency on discharge (Uldall et al. 2000).

In this case, the patient's complicated pharmacopeia likely contributed to his altered mental status. Various suspect medications included anticholinergic agents (scopolamine), opioids (hydromorphone, morphine, fentanyl), and sedatives (zolpidem). Other systemic medical factors likely contributing to his delirium included multiple infections (peritoneal tuberculosis, *Clostridium difficile* colitis, and pneumonia) and metabolic derangements (as evidenced by increased serum ammonia).

The patient's medication regimen was streamlined to the fullest extent possible, infections were diagnosed and treated, hyperammonemia was identified (lactulose was held secondary to a multitude of gastrointestinal problems), and an antipsychotic (olanzapine) was initiated. After most of the causes of delirium were addressed, it was possible to more clearly isolate the hydromorphone as being directly related to the patient's episodic confusion. At this point, donepezil was chosen as a more targeted therapy for the patient's suspected opiate-related delirium (Slatkin and Rhiner 2004; Slatkin et al. 2001). Within several days the patient's MMSE score had returned to 30. His mental status remained stable when olanzapine was discontinued.

Notably, our patient's depression and anxiety may have represented early symptoms of "minor cognitive-motor disorder" or HIV-associated dementia. Formal neuropsychological evaluation (not available in the acute care setting) could help further clarify impairments (Tozzi et al. 2007). He was noted to have abnormalities on head MRI scan, which were read as consistent with either PML or HIV encephalitis. Although the current first-line treatment for PML, HIV encephalitis, and HIV-associated dementia is CART (Berenguer et al. 2003; Clifford et al. 1999), recent studies have shown that cognitive deficits of HIV-associated dementia may not completely resolve with CART (Robertson et al. 2007). Our patient was able to restart CART prior to discharge from the hospital. We consider his resiliency in the face of significant illness and his rapid return to a normal score on the MMSE to be prognostically positive factors.

HIV, Narcissistic Personality Disorder, and Dysthymic disorder

The HIV epidemic had been devastating to individuals and communities alike. Although initially representing a terminal illness with little hope of meaningful recovery and function, it has been transformed by modern treatment methods to a chronic and relapsing illness that requires the patient to adapt to the threat to physical and psychic integrity over time while striving to maintain optimized social function. The effects of this epidemic on groups with disadvantaged social and occupational function are familiar to all clinicians. Less intimately familiar, perhaps, are the effects of living with HIV disease on those who are driven to maintain high function despite this illness. This is a case of a highly accomplished patient with a very high level of social function who developed HIV disease in midlife, hardly the usual stereotype of this illness.

A 53-year-old male executive presented with symptoms of mild depression, neurovegetative signs, and interpersonal loneliness. He had an upbringing featuring a distant, critical father with a significant criminal history; the father had been imprisoned during the patient's youth, and they had had only glancing contact in later years. The patient was an only child and somewhat indulged by his mother, who inculcated in him expectations of high levels of academic and occupational achievement. He was a high achiever in school, and after completing his university degree he then trained as an aviator and had a long and successful career in government service.

He had several assignments overseas where he interfaced with high-ranking officials of host governments. During his spare time, he completed his doctoral degree and also served as an elected official in his community of residence. After his retirement from a government agency, he worked as an executive in the human resources field. He had never married, having been unable to commit to women emotionally, largely due to his focus on his career and other success objects.

He contracted HIV in his 40s after a relationship with a woman in a foreign country, whom he had met while on assignment. He was unaware of her HIV status, and after he contracted HIV he had no further contact with her. In the months after developing HIV, he became mildly depressed, which led him to seek out treatment. He was treated with a serotonin-norepinephrine reuptake inhibitor, with symptomatic improvement. Upon seeking out psychotherapy, his motivation for care was a greater level of self-understanding to deal with his now chronic illness and a desire to become capable of emotional intimacy. Very proud of his high level of intellectual function, and likely reacting to a sense of threat to this from his illness, he related at his clinical intake that he found it "hard to connect to other people." As an illustrative example, he described how he was a member of Mensa and went to Mensa meetings regularly. However, he said that "the other Mensa members are not very interesting to me. I have nothing to talk to them about." Despite living alone (no marriages and no recent intimate relationships), he maintained a set of "50 place settings of fine china, crystal, and silverware, in case I have company." Sadly, he rarely did have guests.

In psychotherapy sessions, he presented as intellectualized, emotionally distant, superior in attitude, and with a tendency to challenge the clinician on an intellectual level. He demanded constant attention during sessions, even bringing a gift of a small clock that he placed on the bookshelf behind the patient's chair "so you won't have to look away from me to look at your watch." His approach to his HIV was similarly narcissistic; he demanded personalized "on-demand" attention from his infectious disease specialist and the specialist's staff; he expected his regular laboratory results to be shared with him in a "collegial" way and wanted detailed discussions about all the parameters of new medications. Not surprisingly, he was fanatical about self-care, exercise, and health maintenance, a point of great pride for him.

◆ **Diagnosis: Axis I—Dysthymic Disorder, 300.4; Axis II— Narcissistic Personality Disorder, 301.81**

Even aside from his HIV status, this patient was a notably high-functioning yet simultaneously vulnerable, lonely, and depressive narcissistic character. His pattern of professional and academic achievement represented "hypersublimation" of interpersonal loneliness and impoverishment. As he approached normative midlife challenges, he was at risk for significant depression because the rewards of his sublimation behavior no longer compensated for his lack of intimacy, his feeling isolated on his island of success, and other narcissistic challenges. At this very time (quite surprisingly, as he did not generally follow a high-risk lifestyle), he contracted HIV disease. Beyond the feeling of anger at his female partner for having infected him, he then had to devote significant energy to disease management, all the while needing to continue his high level of narcissistic achievement. Psychosomatic medicine psychiatrists treating HIV patients of high occupational function should consider the formulation of narcissistic personality disorder, as seen in this man, and tailor their psychotherapeutic approach with an appreciation of the psychiatric aspects of HIV disease.

References

Berenguer J, Miralles P, Arrizabalaga J, et al: Clinical course and prognostic factors of progressive multifocal leukoencephalopathy in patients treated with highly active antiretroviral therapy. Clin Infect Dis 36:1047–1052, 2003

Berger JR, Brew B: An international screening tool for HIV dementia. AIDS 19:2165, 2005

Clifford DB, Yiannoutsos C, Glicksman M, et al: HAART improves prognosis in HIV-associated progressive multifocal leukoencephalopathy. Neurology 52:623–625, 1999

Folstein MF, Folstein SE, McHugh PR: "Mini-Mental State": a practical method for grading the cognitive state of patients for the clinician. J Psychiatr Res 12:189–198, 1975

Klinkenberg WD, Sacks S: Mental disorders and drug abuse in persons living with HIV/AIDS. Aids Care 16:22–42, 2004

Perkins DO, Davidson EJ, Leserman J, et al: Personality disorder in patients infected with HIV: a controlled study with implications for clinical care. Am J Psychiatry 150:309–315, 1993

Reger M, Welsh R, Razani J, et al: A meta-analysis of the neuropsychological sequelae of HIV infection. J Int Neuropsychol Soc 8:410–424, 2002

Robertson KR, Smurzynski M, Pasons TD, et al: The prevalence and incidence of neurocognitive impairment in the HAART era. AIDS 21:1915, 2007

Simpson D: HIV Rounds at Cornell: selected neurologic complications of HIV disease. AIDS Patient Care STDs 12:209–215, 1998

Slatkin N, Rhiner M: Treatment of opiate-induced delirium with acetylcholinesterase inhibitors: a case report. J Pain Symptom Manage 27:268–273, 2004

Slatkin NE, Rhiner M, Bolton TM: Donepezil in the treatment of opioid-induced sedation: a report of six cases. J Pain Symptom Manage 21:425–438, 2001

Tozzi V, Balestra P, Bellagamba R, et al: Persistence of neuropsychologic deficits despite long-term highly active antiretroviral therapy in patients with

HIV-related neurocognitive impairment: prevalence and risk factors. J Acquir Immune Defic Syndr 45:174, 2007

Uldall KK, Harris VL, Lalone B: Outcomes associated with delirium in acutely hospitalized acquired immune deficiency syndrome patients. Compr Psychiatry 41:88, 2000

Walkup J, Crystal S, Sambamoorthi U: Schizophrenia and major affective disorder among Medicaid recipients with HIV/AIDS in New Jersey. Am J Public Health 89:1101–1103, 1999

DERMATOLOGY

The relationship of dermatology and psychosomatic medicine may initially seem a bit indirect. These conditions are generally more chronic than acute and are generally less dramatic and life- threatening than illness affecting other organ systems. Nonetheless, the skin may be the site of self-injury in factitious disorder, there may be dermatologic side effects of central nervous system–active medications, and the skin may be the affected organ system in delusional systems. In addition, severe skin lesions may be associated with reclusiveness and other signs of social avoidance.

Methamphetamine-Induced Skin Excoriations

The patient was a 39-year-old right-handed shift worker in a food processing plant who had weeping and inflamed sores on his skin that were prominent on his left arm, abdomen, face, and legs and had developed over the previous 18 months. He had had an extensive medical workup with particular attention paid to possible allergic causes for what he described as "an itch everywhere in my skin." The lesions were clearly self-induced from gouging at his skin in response to the unbearable sensations he experienced. He had been asked repeatedly whether he believed he had "bugs living in his skin" and whether the sores represented his attempts to "dig them out." He denied feeling as though he were infested. He also denied any obsessive thoughts or rituals suggestive of obsessive-compulsive disorder. The dermatologist who had been prescribing wet wraps and steroid creams with some benefit had given him the diagnoses of neurodermatitis or possible neurotic excoriations and referred him for psychiatric consultation.

The patient denied any previous formal psychiatric history, and there was nothing about his mental status examination suggestive of delusional psychopathology. He did, however, endorse an extensive substance abuse history. He had had several chemical dependency treatments since his late teens for alcohol dependence. Although he was vague about the details, he eventually admitted that he continued to drink on an almost daily basis and used marijuana "when I can get it."

Pushed further, he somewhat defensively revealed that he had experimented with cocaine in the past and more recently had tried methamphetamine. With increasingly persistent questioning, he revealed that "trying meth" actually consisted of having used it every weekend for the past 18 months, a time frame that corresponded exactly with the emergence of his skin lesions. "I never take it when I'm going to work," he said, "but I like to kick back on the weekends with my girlfriend."

Although he considered himself to be a "recreational user," he recognized that there was a clear connection between the onset of his methamphetamine use and the eruption of the skin sores. With prodding from the dermatologist and the psychiatrist, he agreed to enter a residential drug treatment program, and over the several weeks he was there the skin lesions resolved completely, only to recur soon after his discharge.

◆ **Diagnosis: Axis I—Polysubstance Dependence, 304.80**

This case underscores the differential diagnosis of psychiatric causes of dermatologic lesions, including delusional parasitosis, obsessive-compulsive picking, and drug-induced formication (Dunn et al. 2007). The true cause only emerged after persistent and empathic questioning by the psychiatric consultant. The rehabilitation period allowed a "natural history" of healing to emerge while the patient was in the process of substance dependence recovery. Sadly, the prompt recurrence of the lesions thereafter correlates with recurrence of his methamphetamine use.

Factitious Disorder With Dermatological Ulceration

A 62-year-old retired psychiatric nurse prompted a psychiatric consultation request from the dermatology service after she had been evaluated by neurologists, vascular and plastic surgeons, and infectious disease and rheumatology specialists. She was admitted to the medical center after two prior evaluations at distant tertiary care facilities for a nonhealing erosive lesion at the hairline on her right forehead. The patient said it all began with an insect bite at a family reunion 2 years earlier. Initial swelling and pruritis gave way to a firm lump that eventually began to weep serous fluid and, later, frank pus. The margins of the lesion gradually widened, leaving the patient with a quarter-sized ulceration 6 months after the initial bite. A succession of topical remedies either provided brief or minimal evidence of improvement. The patient was hospitalized once for intensive wound care over a 2-week period. The margins of the wound began to appear healthier as granulation tissue appeared in the ulcerative crater. Over subsequent months, however, the ulceration deepened and erosion of the skull became apparent. By the time of the patient's admission to the dermatology service, the erosion had penetrated her skull.

An intelligent woman, the patient was able to give an excellent description of factitious disorder although she insisted that she had never manipulated the wound. Her husband, also a mental health professional, confirmed that he had never had reason to doubt her denial of a factitial component. Nonetheless, a careful psychosocial review uncovered a succession of corrosive stresses in the patient's life.

About 3 years prior to admission, the patient's only daughter had committed suicide after a tumultuous decade of polysubstance abuse punctuated by periodic phases of sobriety, all of which followed treatment programs arranged by the patient and her husband. The patient's son-in-law, never a consistent presence in the marriage, vanished and left the care of their three children in the hands of the patient. She described the younger two children in glowing terms but was curiously silent about the oldest, a teenage girl.

The patient's resistance to discussing this adolescent aroused the psychiatry consultant's interest. Persistent probing eventually yielded an animated account of the havoc this child had introduced to the family. Frequently truant from school, drawn to a provocative circle of friends, disrespectful of family boundaries and in recurring difficulty with the law, this hyperactive adolescent seemed to have successfully commandeered the central role in the household. Whereas the patient had been accustomed to enjoying the undivided attention of her husband, a prominent place in local society, and the pleasure of frequent travel, she now increasingly found herself expending enormous energy and time reacting to the continuous challenges kicked up by her granddaughter's behavior. Nor could she muster sustained anger in response, because she realized that the child's mother and then her father had both essentially abandoned the children.

It was in this vexed context that the patient developed the progressive lesion on her forehead and discovered that it procured an incremental restoration of important elements of her prior life. Successive evaluations at ever more distant tertiary care medical centers became the studied objective of her caring husband. He arranged for expensive childcare and accompanied her to various cities for multiple consultations. Friends who had shunned her when the granddaughter's behavior was strewn about the local community's gossip networks now rallied to commiserate over her cryptic medical affliction. Curiously, she said she did not mind having had to surrender her passion for swimming, adding that the turban-like bandage she wore elicited frequent and kind sympathy from neighbors and strangers alike. Even her granddaughter seemed to have found the wherewithal to temper her behavior somewhat; perhaps aware at some level that the potential outcome of a lesion that had succeeded in perforating bone was not benign.

◆ **Diagnosis: Axis I—Factitious Disorder With Predominantly Physical Signs and Symptoms, 300.19**

Suffering was no stranger to this patient. The parent of an only child, she watched her daughter's promising future succumb to the repeated assaults of addiction. She and her husband invested love, time, and ever-larger sums of money in extended treatment programs. Hope was kindled over and again, only to be extinguished by the next relapse. She wanted to believe that the three children would provide her daughter with the elusive incentive to maintain sobriety. The patient knew the resonant tension with which her daughter had lived. Years of surrogate anxiety depleted her emotional reserves and painted the prospect of retirement and travel with her husband with deep appeal. The loss of her daughter to suicide and the loss of retirement to a second parental commitment turned her world upside down.

The demands of caring for three children who struggled with their own unique demons of bereavement exhausted the patient. Her husband found some solace in his medical practice while the patient abruptly resigned from her position to make time for the children and, in so doing, lost important sources of adult companionship and support. The forehead lesion became a road to connection, caring, and control.

Reference

Dunn J, Murphy MB, Fox KM: Diffuse pruritic lesions in a 37-year-old man after sleeping in an abandoned building. Am J Psychiatry 164:1166–1172, 2007

12

SURGERY

The surgery services in medical centers are the source of some of the more dramatic and tragic patient stories and the place for some of the most important interventions in psychosomatic medicine. The dramatic nature of many surgical problems, the fact that surgical patients must frequently confront life-or-death situations, the risks for delirium in surgical patients, and other factors make the interaction with surgical services one of the more common and critical areas of psychosomatic medicine. Whether one is dealing with postoperative delirium, assessing decisional capacity for surgical informed consent, or helping patients and family members deal with bad news, the surgical services require a great many psychosomatic medicine interventions.

A Case of Family Illness and Evolving Symptoms

A 52-year-old Asian American man woke with severe pain in his throat, which radiated up his neck, down his back, and into his lower extremities. After 7 hours of efforts to resolve the pain (including resting, eating, acetaminophen, and ibuprofen), the patient presented to a community hospital, where he was found to have an acute type A aortic dissection. The patient was rapidly transferred to a university medical center for emergent surgery. He did well when extubated on postoperative day 2 and was transferred out of the surgical intensive care unit to a telemetry unit. Within 12 hours of transfer, the patient became notably anxious and restless. He was treated with a total of 30 mg of lorazepam, 8 mg of morphine, and 4 mg haloperidol, all with little effect.

The psychosomatic medicine service was called to evaluate this patient for suspected alcohol withdrawal on the morning of postoperative day 3. At this point the patient was intermittently agitated, diaphoretic, tremulous, mildly hypertensive (blood pressure 130–

146 mm Hg/74–88 mm Hg), and tachycardic (93–111 beats per minute). He did not answer any questions coherently. Prior to surgery, the patient had given variable reports of the amount he drank to different surgery resident physicians managing his care—ranging from "four beers a couple of times a week" to "18 beers on occasion." Collateral information from his wife was equally questionable; she reported that the patient had drunk since they were married 15 years ago, "but it never was a problem." She also reported that the patient had no past psychiatric history and that he was a high-functioning small business owner and held a local political office.

The patient was transferred back to the intensive care unit and started on an intravenous lorazepam drip, which was rapidly titrated up to 7 mg/hour. The patient continued to demonstrate autonomic instability and agitation, which was particularly risky given his recent aortic repair. On postoperative day 4, the patient was reintubated and started on a propofol drip. He remained heavily sedated for 2 days, switching from propofol to midazolam drip and eventually to diazepam 10 mg every 4 hours. Olanzapine, orally dissolving tablets, 5 mg twice daily was added for agitation and delirium. The patient was reextubated on postoperative day 6 but remained confused and unable to communicate; his Mini-Mental State Examination (MMSE; Folstein et al. 1975) score was 0. Metoprolol, hydralazine, and clonidine were recommended by cardiology because of his high blood pressure (140–167 mm Hg/66–119 mm Hg) and tachycardia (98–109 beats per minute), which persisted even while the patient appeared quite sedated. A thorough workup for other causes of delirium, including cultures for infectious sources, thyroid-stimulating hormone levels, complete blood cell count, chemistry panels, NH_3, and liver-associated enzymes was negative. The patient received very few opioids during this time, so this was not considered a significant contributor to his altered mental status.

The patient continued to have a complicated hospital course; he remained poorly communicative until postoperative day 10, at which point his MMSE score had improved to 21 and his vital signs had stabilized (blood pressure 95–113 mm Hg/54–77 mm Hg; heart rate 93–99 beats per minute). On his 12th hospital day, the psychosomatic medicine service was called for an emergent decisional capacity evaluation when the patient was trying to leave against medical advice. At this point, he was still being closely monitored for his blood pressure, and his multiple antihypertensives were not all yet transitioned from intravenous to oral forms. The psychiatry resident on call, called in to see the patient emergently, noted the patient to have rapid speech, labile mood, and grandiosity. His MMSE score remained at 21, and the patient demonstrated limited understanding of the seriousness of his medical condition; as such, he did not demonstrate adequate decisional capacity to sign himself out. The patient was thought to still be delirious, and an underlying mood disorder was also suspected. His wife, acting as surrogate decision maker under the circumstances of his decisional capacity deficit, consented for his ongoing treatment.

The patient's residual delirium appeared to clear over the next few days (on day 15, his MMSE score was 26), and diazepam was tapered and discontinued. At this point, because his cognitive status had improved significantly, the patient was interviewed in greater detail regarding his alcohol consumption and past psychiatric history. He admitted to years of mood swings characterized by increased sociability and productivity alternating with periods of profound anhedonia. This was in keeping with the observation made by the psychosomatic medicine service that as his cognition improved the patient was noted to be overly social with hospital staff, with loud, rapid speech and grandiosity of thought content. It remained unclear what relationship alcohol played in these mood swings. A provisional diagnosis of bipolar disorder not otherwise specified was added to his formulation. Olanzapine was increased to 10 mg twice a day for mood instability.

In regard to alcohol abuse, the patient gave positive responses to three out of the four CAGE questions. Interestingly, he noted that although he may have drunk too much in the past, he believed it was really his "wife who had the problem" (complaints about his wife endangering their child by drinking heavily while caring for the child had previously resulted in a child protective services report). Having identified that the patient was at the "precontemplative" stage of change regarding his motivation to examine his pattern of alcohol consumption (Prochaska and DiClemente 1992; Prochaska et al. 1992), the service presented the patient with the evidence that in fact he had suffered serious physical disability (prolonged stay in intensive care with reintubation) substantially secondary to his alcohol use. Despite these efforts, at the end of his 17-day hospitalization the patient invited hospital personnel to an alcohol-themed party (which he called a "kegger") to celebrate his recovery.

◆ **Diagnosis: Axis I—Alcohol Dependence, 303.90; Alcohol Withdrawal, 291.81; Bipolar Disorder Not Otherwise Specified, 296.80; Delirium (Resolved) 293.0; Axis II—Narcissistic Traits, Rule Out Narcissistic Personality Disorder, 301.81**

Alcohol withdrawal is a common and potentially very serious problem seen in hospitalized patients. Unrecognized or severe alcohol withdrawal can result in seizures, autonomic instability, agitation, and delirium tremens (DTs). These complications are especially dangerous in the medically ill. Accurately determining a patient's risk for withdrawal/DTs can be challenging. Patients frequently underestimate or actively misrepresent the amount of alcohol they consume. Trauma patients may present with altered mental status and an inability to give any history. Family-provided collateral information, while often desirable, is not always reliable.

The diagnosis of alcohol dependence/withdrawal in a patient with an unclear consumption history is frequently based on circumstantial evidence. A number of factors may help in making a diagnosis. Mental status examination may be characterized by the classic tremulousness, diaphoresis, agitation, and vital sign instability. Although blood alcohol level is often undetectable by the time alcohol withdrawal is suspected, indirect indicators of alcohol dependence may include elevated mean corpuscular volume, aspartate aminotransferase, γ-glutamyltransferase, carbohydrate-deficient transferrin, and homocysteine and/or decreased folate and magnesium.

Another difficulty in diagnosing alcohol withdrawal in medically ill patients is that multiple systemic comorbidities and medications may contribute to delirium. In a case such as the one just described, a postoperative patient is susceptible to infections, lingering effects of anesthetic agents, and opioids. Although the conservative approach dictates erring on the side of overdiagnosing and thus overtreating for alcohol withdrawal, the benzodiazepines we use to treat this condition can have exacerbating effects on delirium from other causes. Another difficult decision involves the use of antipsychotic medications in cases of suspected alcohol withdrawal. Although atypical antipsychotics can be quite helpful in delirium due to other etiologies, in cases of alcohol withdrawal, antipsychotics have been found to worsen autonomic instability and may lower the seizure threshold.

Effective treatment for alcohol withdrawal results in improvement in autonomic instability, prevention of seizures, and the alleviation of the physical discomfort of withdrawal states. Most cases can be treated effectively with short- or long-acting benzodiazepines administered according to a variety of protocols. Other medications that have been shown to be helpful in the treatment of alcohol withdrawal include propofol and phenobarbital, but the use of these medications is limited by their relatively narrow "therapeutic index" and frequent need for intubation. In our case, controlling the patient's elevated blood pressure and heart rate was of paramount importance, and the decision to move from benzodiazepines to propofol/intubation was made by an intensivist based on the high-risk situation that the patient was postoperative from an aortic dissection repair. Only after alcohol withdrawal was well controlled was the patient extubated and transitioned to a long-acting benzodiazepine (diazepam).

Substance abuse, mood disorder, and personality disorder are not an uncommon triad in patients presenting with serious illness or injury. The treatment of patients with this combination of synergistic psychopathology is challenging in a psychiatric setting, and possibly more so when defenses are at their most primitive during a hospital stay. This case was unusual in the degree of denial seemingly demonstrated by both the patient and his wife; they both minimized the amount of alcohol the patient consumed, the severity of mood instability, and the seriousness of the pain the patient presented with. This case demonstrates how family dynamics may work to contain/enable pathology until a crisis reveals the extent of family dysfunction. This patient likely had many years of undiagnosed bipolar disorder and alcohol dependence that had been tolerated by an equally disabled spouse.

Acute Penile Laceration:
A Case of Changing Attribution

A 44-year-old single white man presented to the emergency department of a university medical center with a penile laceration and "8 out of 10" pain. The patient initially stated that he woke up the morning of presentation with a laceration on his penis after having sexual intercourse with a woman he did not know well. He assumed that the woman cut his penis before leaving his home. He had presented for care when he noted his urine was leaking from the shaft of his penis. After emergency department physicians observed that the laceration appeared in fact to be several days old, the patient revised his story, reporting that he had an episode of priapism which he tried to remedy himself with a kitchen knife.

Psychosomatic medicine psychiatry was initially consulted to assess the patient's decisional capacity to consent to surgery for urethral repair and insertion of a suprapubic catheter. The patient gave a history of schizoaffective disorder and alcohol dependence, and the primary surgery team was concerned that the patient's mental illness might interfere with his ability to understand the risks and benefits of surgery. The patient appeared to understand his medical condition quite well and wanted to proceed with the proposed surgery; his MMSE score was 27. The patient stated his psychiatric symptoms were adequately managed with quetiapine 100 mg at bedtime, olanzapine 20 mg and paroxetine 60 mg orally every morning, and chlordiazepoxide 25 mg three times a day, although he associated the reported priapism with the recent addition of quetiapine to his medication regimen. He refused permission for contact with his outpatient psychiatrist or family members, noting that he was an "extremely intelligent person" and could tell the psychosomatic medicine psychiatrists "whatever they needed to know" about his past psychiatric history. He was found to have intact decisional capacity to accept the proposed urological surgery.

The patient and psychosomatic medicine team developed greater rapport over the next several days, and eventually the patient gave a third accounting of his penile laceration. He admitted that the previously shared stories about the woman cutting him and about the priapism were untrue. He now described experiencing persecutory auditory hallucinations prior to his cutting himself that had convinced him that he "should be a woman." He had attempted to cut off his penis to follow the commands of the auditory hallucinations. The patient immediately regretted his action but delayed receiving medical attention due to his embarrassment over his act. Suspecting a possible gender identity disorder, the psychiatry resident inquired about the patient perhaps having had lifelong feelings of being the wrong gender and discomfort with his genitalia. The patient fervently denied these feelings, noting that up until the day of the incident he had felt quite comfortable with his gender identity.

During his hospital stay, the patient needed several surgical procedures to reconstruct his urethra, and he required skin grafting and placement of a suprapubic catheter. The patient's psychotropic medications were managed, and he was counseled on alcohol cessation. The patient's mother came to the hospital and, now with consent of the patient, gave the psychosomatic medicine service more information about his developmental history. She noted that the patient had previously been an excellent student and had earned a graduate degree; however, tragically he had had his first psychotic episode while in his late 20s and working as an engineer.

She reported having tried many times to assist him with managing his finances and housing and with obtaining help for his substance abuse. However, she reported feeling helpless in these attempts because he often rejected her offers of assistance. Prior to discharge from the medical center, the patient agreed to a telephone conference with the psychosomatic medicine team and his outpatient psychiatrist to discuss what had occurred and to ensure close outpatient psychiatric care. Rapid follow-up was arranged, and the patient was discharged back to home with his suprapubic catheter still in place.

◆ **Diagnosis: Axis I—Schizoaffective Disorder, Bipolar Type, 295.70; Alcohol Dependence, 303.90; Axis II—Narcissistic Personality Traits**

This patient presented with a striking combination of influential auditory hallucinations, impulsivity, and sufficient insight to "cover up" some of his more disturbing psychiatric symptoms. The psychiatric consult on this patient was initially called for an assessment of decisional capacity for him to consent to surgery. Although the patient had demonstrated markedly poor judgment prior to presentation to the hospital, he had no significant cognitive impairment or psychotic symptoms that interfered with his rational consideration of the proposed surgical procedure at the time of this clinical evaluation. In fact, the patient showed little evidence of overtly psychotic symptoms during his 2-week admission. However, his act of genital self-mutilation was so disturbing to the various medical care providers that the patient's subsequent ability to make *any* medical decisions was repeatedly called into question.

This case invites an exploration of the psychodynamics behind such a self-mutilative act. A psychoanalytic view of the content of this patient's psychotic symptoms suggests a deep discomfort with overwhelming sexual and aggressive impulses. The patient's auditory hallucinations may have represented unconscious guilty feelings regarding virility, leading the patient to his attempted autocastration. Alternatively, given his mother's ongoing attempts to provide aid and comfort to the patient well into adulthood, the patient's actions may have represented a desire to circumvent emasculation by her, rather than continuously fearing attacks on his masculinity.

On a more concrete level, the psychosomatic medicine team regarded the later-repudiated story shared by this patient regarding priapism as feasible, given emerging evidence in case report literature that quetiapine can be associated with this side effect in therapeutic doses and overdose (Davol and Rukstalis 2005; Harrison et al. 2006; Pais and Ayvazia 2001). The patient's ongoing alcohol use was also regarded as an important contributor to his impulsivity and a target for future therapy, although it remained unclear whether the patient was drinking alcohol at the time he cut himself. Finally, the patient's narcissistic personality traits appeared to hinder his ability to seek care when he needed it, while his guardedness served to keep healthcare providers from communicating with each other. The team affirmed the patient's autonomy in medical decision making and was pleased by the patient's efforts to secure his own psychiatric follow-up.

Burns, Delirium, and Posttraumatic Stress Disorder

The environment of the burn surgery unit offers a cornucopia of psychopathology (van der Does et al. 1997). Common psychiatric diagnoses among burn patients are delirium, substance abuse disorders, and acute stress disorder (ASD).

> The patient was a 45-year-old man who worked as a welder on an oil pipeline. An explosion occurred during a welding job, killing the patient's work companion and causing the patient severe burns. He was urgently admitted to the burn unit for surgical care. For the first several days of hospitalization he was profoundly delirious, with altered sleep-wake cycle, agitation, decreased cognitive function, and variable mental status. His delirium was likely exacerbated by the regular use of intravenous opioids and midazolam for frequent, painful burn dressing changes. He was managed with risperidone, with some improvement in sleep-wake cycle and cognition and with less agitation.
>
> Several days after his initial improvement, be became acutely agitated one night, screamed that he had to "get away from the fire," and crawled out of his bed, putting his dressings and burn wounds at risk. He was actively reexperiencing the precipitating event of his trauma, something he had heretofore been unable to recall on earlier interviews while he was being managed for delirium. He was subsequently put on mirtazapine (in addition to continuing risperi-

done) with subsequent better sleep, no further nightmares, and no more agitated behavior.

♦ **Diagnosis: Axis I—Posttraumatic Stress Disorder, 309.81; Delirium, 293.0**

This case dramatically illustrates two important and related points. First, owing to the nature of severe burns, with the attendant risk for dehydration and infection, severely burned patients are at high risk for the development of delirium. In addition, the surgical management of burns (lengthy and frequent surgery, and often more-than-once-daily dressing changes with premedication using intravenous opioids and benzodiazepines) is a medical management model that is itself highly delirium prone. In addition, burn patients often acquire significant infections that require infection control isolation, which diminishes the amount of contact they have with visitors, nurses, and other staff members.

The risk of acute stress disorder (ASD)/posttraumatic stress disorder (PTSD) must always be actively considered in these patients. By the very nature of severe burns, they are *a priori* a severely life-threatening event. In addition, the physical environmental context of many severe burns, including physical trauma and other life-threatening injuries, increases the risk of ASD/PTSD as well. Somewhat less dramatic but important to consider is the sense of retraumatization at the hands of physicians and nurses who must regularly expose the patient to painful and traumatizing medical and surgical interventions.

This patient's onset of ASD was significantly delayed following the accident that caused his burns. Initially, while delirious, he was significantly cognitively impaired in the context of delirium and was not able to recall this accident. However, with treatment of delirium and improved cognitive status, he was able to begin to remember his accident and to become in touch with the experience, including the death of his coworker, who was also a close friend. In that context, he developed many of the symptoms of ASD, which, once recognized and treated, responded well to routine treatment with the sedating antidepressant mirtazapine (which was added to the risperidone initially given for delirium).

Psychosomatic medicine psychiatrists treating trauma victims with an initial presentation of delirium should be alert to the possibility of "tardive acute stress disorder" as described in this case. An explanatory model to consider is that the acute delirium, which is conceptualized as a temporary imbalance among acetylcholine, dopamine, and perhaps other neurotransmitters, "suspends" the cognitive processing of traumatic memories. Perhaps some patients are only temporarily amnestic for these memories owing to acute delirium; once the delirium is managed, the memory circuitry (presumably invoking a hippocampal mechanism) can then restore more normal function, including awareness of traumatic stimuli.

The other aspect to consider is that of a "two-stage" model of ASD/PTSD. The first stage is the initial physical trauma resulting in the severe injury. Somewhat more obscure, however, is the second-stage trauma, which is caused by painful and physically threatening medical and surgical procedures. The psychosomatic medicine consultant should be willing to address medical and surgical interventions as traumatic events when processing the overall trauma experience of these unfortunate patients.

It can be difficult to distinguish motor agitation due to delirium from motor agitation due to ASD—for example, in the setting of nightmares or flashbacks. Although the distinction may not be absolute, several points of departure exist. Agitation due to ASD will often be episodic and temporally associated with current experiences of flashbacks or nightmares. ASD patients will typically have an anxious appearance and be otherwise largely cognitively intact. The nightmares and flashbacks of ASD (as opposed to those of delirium) typically have themes relating to the traumatic experience (either real or symbolic), while the perceptual disturbances driving delirium agitation may be more random in nature. In burn patients, psychosomatic medicine physicians may thus be alert to the possible sequence of psychiatric complication of "delirium early, ASD later."

"There Is a Gerbil Eating My Foot"

Misattribution of sensory stimuli, technically an illusion rather than a true hallucination, may be seen in hospitalized patients, especially in the context of delirium and serious illness or injury. Patients with baseline poor socialization and poor coping skills may be particularly prone to such misattributions, although this connection may be difficult to establish causally.

> The patient was a 35-year-old single white man. He had, at baseline, an isolated lifestyle (no intimate partnerships, a propensity for solitary activity, and low educational and occupational achievement). He eked out a meager living as a professional "dog walker" (he would temporarily care for the pets of clients while the clients traveled) in a major city. He had not had a formal psychiatric evaluation before presenting to the hospital. He attended a gathering where one of the participant activities was to walk barefoot over hot coals in a kind of a "cleansing" ritual. While doing this activity, he sustained serious burns to both feet and needed admission to the burn unit.
>
> On interview, his solitary lifestyle and tendency toward eccentric attributions and other behaviors were felt to be consistent with schizotypal traits versus personality disorder. He explained in a rather idiosyncratic fashion that since the name of the gathering was the "Burning Man" festival (an annual event in Nevada), he felt the "burning" of his feet was somehow cleansing to him; hence his excessive exposure to the burning coals, leading to his injuries.
>
> The next evening he became agitated and began to struggle to remove the dressing and bandage from one of his feet. He had awakened from a dream agitated and began to scream about a "large gerbil" that was "eating" his foot. He described the gerbil as "big, white, and fluffy," and, gesturing, he pointed to the dressing and bandage as representing the "gerbil." Because it was critical to his recovery that he not interfere with the integrity of the dressing and bandage, he was treated with a low dose of risperidone. With treatment, he was able to correctly understand that the bandage was not in fact threatening him, and he subsequently did well, had no further delusional misattributions, recovered, and was eventually sent home.

◆ **Diagnosis: Axis I—Delirium, 293.0; Axis II—Schizotypal Personality Disorder, 301.22**

Psychotic misattribution of a medical device as another foreign object led this man to become agitated and to threaten his dressing, ultimately putting his physical recovery at risk. Prompt use of antipsychotic medication and active feedback to support accurate reality testing led to his being able to give up the illusion. Psychosomatic medicine psychiatrists should be alert to such delusional misattributions, especially in patients in intensive care units, where innocuous medical materials may be subject to delusional misidentification, with resultant increases in already significant levels of patient distress.

Narcissistic Personality Disorder, Dramatic Suicidality, and Overattachment

The combination of severe personality disorder, medically complicated severe suicide attempts, and maladaptive coping behavior to the consequences of suicidal acts is a potent one. In dramatic cases, it is associated with significant consumption of medical and surgical resources. Treatment of these patients requires patience, persistence, and an ability to manage severe personality pathology.

> The patient was a 50-year-old man with a history of episodic depression. He was also morbidly obese, weighing more than 400 pounds. He had no significant interpersonal relationships; his only close attachment figure, his mother, had died several months previously. He was estranged from his father, who actively disowned him when finally located by a resourceful social worker. He had never married and had no children. In the context of the depression over his mother's death, he had made an escalating series of suicide attempts, after which he would present to the emergency department for medical care. Each attempt was more life threatening than the previous one. He presented to the emergency department yet again seeking psychiatric care. After being told he was not going to be sent to a psychiatric facility, he went into the department's men's room and, with a large knife, stabbed himself in the midline.
>
> His injuries included a puncture of the right ventricle and a deep midline abdominal wound that extended to the umbilicus. After emergency trauma surgery to repair his heart and his abdomen, he was admitted to the intensive care unit. After surgical recovery, a psychosomatic medicine consultation was accomplished. Upon interview, he said that he was no longer suicidal "because since I injured myself, now people understand how badly I have been feeling." He was, however, still severely depressed. His unresolved grief for his mother was overwhelming. He described an enmeshed relationship with her in which "we would do everything together." His obesity was promoted by his and his mother's daily large meals together, conducted in a ritualistic fashion. He did not know what to do without her and actively spoke of wishing to be reunited with her "in heaven" as motivating his escalating suicide attempts. He was also grandiose and self-referential and felt entitled to special treatment. He was treated with an antidepressant and followed closely.

Shortly after his initial stabilization, he had brief period of cardiac arrest and was resuscitated. After recovery, he exhibited mild cognitive impairment (suggesting mild hypoxic injury) and was now, in addition to his baseline narcissistic personality disorder and depression, inattentive and disinhibited as well. Because of slow recovery from the surgical injury due to his extreme obesity, he developed a series of decubitus ulcers, many of which required surgical management. He was also felt to be still at significant risk of self-harm in view of his history of serious attempts, ongoing depression, personality disorder, and now behavioral disinhibition. As a result of all of these problems, he had a prolonged hospital course of nearly 1 year.

Late in the hospital course, after an initial period of hostile attachment and entitled, demanding behavior, he now had become pathologically attached to the medical center. This took the form of some extreme, even bordering on bizarre, statements such as, "The trauma unit is like heaven on earth. Where else would anyone want to live?"; "I want to live here forever. Why can't I just move in?"; and "The nurses here, they are like angels." When he was finally surgically cleared, he was sent to inpatient psychiatry for stabilization.

◆ **Diagnosis: Axis I—Major Depressive Disorder, Recurrent, Severe Without Psychotic Features, 296.33; Delirium, 293.0; Axis II—Narcissistic Personality Disorder, 301.81**

The main problem in managing this man was his severe narcissistic personality disorder. He was initially suicidal as a result of profound narcissistic disturbance, loss of interpersonal attachment, and fears of abandonment. Thereafter, his behavior was entitled and demanding. Finally, after attachment to the hospital had been established, he became as pathologically enmeshed with the medical center as he had been with his mother. This illustrates how narcissistic patients, once attached to relationships, can become extremely, even absurdly, dependent on those relationships, even to the point of overlap with dependent personality disorder. Indeed, finally discharging this man had the flavor of "birthing" him to a new institution.

Self-Mutilation Following Delusions

The patient was a 25-year-old single Asian man with a several-year history of schizophrenia. He had a history of psychiatric hospitalization and treatment with various antipsychotics. Despite the use of a psychosocial treatment model in the local county mental health system, the patient was variably noncompliant with psychotropic medication, and his psychotic symptoms persisted. These symptoms included both delusions that he was an "evil person," who had done nonspecific bad things to harm others, and command auditory hallucinations to harm himself in various ways as compensation for his past "evil" behaviors. He was unemployed, reclusive, and minimally socially interactive.

He also developed a most curious dietary delusion. He had come to believe that nearly all food items were contaminated and that if he ate any of them, he would die. Over several months, his list of forbidden foods expanded exponentially to the point that he was eating nothing but cantaloupe for a period of 2 months. It was unclear why cantaloupe remained the only "safe" food.

He was admitted to the medical center with bilateral self-inflicted puncture wounds to the eyes. He had been told by the command hallucinations to "poke his eyes out" to make amends for his past nonspecific "evil" behavior. Because he was not a religious person, this command was not believed to have been based in the distortion of a religious construct. He was urgently taken to ophthalmic surgery, where the right globe was ruptured and vision could not be salvaged. Fortunately, the left eye was surgically repaired and he was able to recover functional vision.

When the psychosomatic medicine service evaluated this patient, he was remarkably calm and unconcerned about his vision loss, stating that he had "had to" follow the directions of the command hallucinations. Preoperatively, he was kept on constant one-to-one watch, because he was both a flight risk and a risk for continued self-harm. Following surgical recovery, he was committed to the county mental health facility because of danger to self and grave disability.

◆ **Diagnosis: Axis I—Schizophrenia, Paranoid Type, 295.30**

This case represented both extreme self-mutilation in response to a command hallucination, with permanent partial functional impairment, and a remarkable food exclusion delusion. It was not clear why cantaloupe remained a "safe" food, because the patient did not appear to have a symbolic connection to this particular food item. This case illustrates the serious risk of self-mutilating behavior in nontreated psychotic states. Behavioral management, both pre- and postoperatively, of patients who self-mutilate during psychotic states must include close behavioral observation against further or repeated self-harm while in the nonpsychiatric medical setting.

Auto-Orchiectomy

The patient was a middle-aged single white man who had recurrent painful epididymitis. He was also uninsured and unemployed, without regular access to healthcare. Following yet another episode of epididymitis, he removed the affected testicle with an X-Acto knife and presented to the medical center with bleeding at the "operative" site. Psychosomatic medicine was consulted due to fears of psychosis or self-mutilation behavior. Upon examination, there was no evidence of psychotic thought process or self-mutilation. He had no formal psychiatric history. He did not express regret over having removed the testis, citing the pain that he had experienced and stating that he had done this solely because he did not have access to regular care. He was otherwise not felt to represent a danger to himself and was not sent to a psychiatric inpatient facility.

♦ **Diagnosis: Axis I—Adjustment Disorder Unspecified, 309.9**

This case illustrates how some acts of self-harm, although clearly representing less than optimal judgment, may be driven by symptoms (persistent pain) and social issues (unemployment and lack of regular medical care) rather than the "usual suspects" of psychotic disorder, mood disorder, or borderline personality disorder. Clearly, this same self-injury could be plausibly connected to psychosis (e.g., based on the belief that the testis represented sinful impulses and thus needed to be removed in a "retributional" or compensatory way) or as a manifestation of borderline personality disorder (angry self-directed harm in the context of abandonment and/or extreme self-loathing). Clinical evaluation by the psychosomatic medicine team was critical in elucidating these factors.

"Cystoscopic Frogectomy"

Surgical services are occasionally called upon to creatively manage the physical consequences of bizarre self-mutilation behavior in psychiatric patients. This is a case of a patient with fetal alcohol syndrome (FAS) and impaired cognitive function who, while distressed, inserted a foreign object through his urethra into his bladder.

A 22-year-old man with FAS presented emergently with fever, chills, anorexia, and dysuria. Examination revealed a metal chain protruding from his urethra. The patient was transferred to a university medical center for urological intervention. An abdominal film and pelvic computed tomography (CT) scans revealed a metal chain in the urethra and a small mass within his bladder. The patient was taken to the operating room, and cystoscopy was performed. A metal chain was removed from the patient's urethra and a plastic toy frog was retrieved from the bladder. Urine cultures showed growth of *Escherichia coli*. He was started on antibiotics for a genitourinary tract infection. A head CT scan revealed microcephaly.

The psychosomatic medicine team was consulted. The patient could not remember the events immediately prior to his hospitalization. Historical information was gathered from his adoptive mother. He had been removed from the care of his biological mother for maternal substance abuse and neglect and was placed in an adoptive family. His youngest sister, who was also diagnosed with FAS, was adopted by the same family. Unlike the patient, the sister had a habit of self-injurious behavior in the form of head banging. In addition to FAS, the patient was diagnosed with attention deficit disorder and had received psychostimulants since the age of 12. Neuropsychological assessments results were obtained, which revealed a verbal IQ of 64 and a performance IQ of 78, yielding a full-scale IQ of 67.

The patient reported being verbally and physically abused by their estranged adoptive father. His adoptive parents had separated 7 months prior to his hospitalization. The patient had destroyed various personal items that were given to him by his foster father. A month prior to the hospitalization, he contemplated suicide by cutting his wrists, hoping that his death would "hurt" his foster father. Two weeks prior to the incident, the patient had become more withdrawn and reclusive. It was during that time, he reported, that he had inserted the toy frog into his own urethra, again hoping that the act of self-harm would hurt the foster father.

His foster mother reported that the patient had the most trouble with social isolation, withdrawal, and irritability. On examination, he had significant microcephaly and an elongated jaw. He was not suicidal, depressed, or experiencing command hallucinations. He had no prior history of self-mutilation. Risperidone 0.5 mg twice daily was started. After recovery, he was discharged to his home with outpatient psychiatric follow-up.

◆ **Diagnosis: Axis I—Attention-Deficit/Hyperactivity Disorder Not Otherwise Specified, 314.9; Axis II—Mild Mental Retardation, 317**

FAS is a leading identifiable cause of mental retardation and neu-rological deficit. Children with FAS may present with comorbid psy-chiatric illness including attention-deficit/hyperactivity, anxiety, mood, conduct, and other behavioral disorders and learning disabil-ities. Self-injurious behavior is also reported. The etiology of self-mutilation is still poorly understood. Self-mutilation is empirically classified into three clinically useful phenomenological categories. One type, characterized by infrequent acts of severe tissue damage, such as eye enucleation, is most often associated with psychosis. The stereotypic type of self-mutilation is monotonously repetitive and rhythmic, such as head-banging, which is often associated with men-tal retardation. Superficial/moderate type self-mutilation is charac-terized by episodic and repetitive behavior such as cutting, often also associated with borderline personality disorder.

Unlike the stereotypic self-injurious behavior generally observed in the mentally retarded, the nature of this patient's self-mutilation is best typed as a unique major episode. It is plausible that the patient may have had a brief episode of psychosis induced by family stres-sors. Although the patient's conscious motive of injuring his penis to injure his father may be explained as delusional, there was no other evidence that the patient was psychotic at the time he acted.

A psychological model in which self-mutilation is employed as a primitive and maladaptive coping mechanism for anxiolysis may apply. The patient was disrupted by the abandonment of his foster father. The patient's inability to recall much of the history surround-ing the event and his experience of childhood abuse support this ex-planation, because he may have mutilated himself during a period of dissociation. Regardless of the explanation, our patient had signifi-cant psychosocial stress, mental retardation, FAS, and a history of abuse. Although children with FAS, like those who are developmen-tally delayed in general, are at risk for stereotyped self-injurious be-havior, this case demonstrates conditions in which major self-mutilation may occur.

Psychosomatic medicine psychiatrists seeing patients with a his-tory of self-mutilation, which may typically be encountered on sur-gical services due to the "surgical" nature of the presenting clinical problem, should consider a wide range of psychopathology in the genesis of these events. Borderline personality disorder and psychotic disorders may be more immediately thought of, but mental retardation and other illnesses characterized by cognitive impairment, especially with behavioral impulsivity and disinhibition in the context of insoluble social stressors, may also be implicated.

Priapism Associated With Risperidone

A rare event in psychiatry is iatrogenic priapism associated with the antidepressant trazodone. However, psychiatrists frequently caution patients against this possibility before initiating treatment with trazodone. Although the association of other psychotropic medications with priapism is probably even more rare, the psychosomatic medicine psychiatrist needs to be alert to this possibility. We present a case of a patient with risperidone-associated priapism, reminding one to be vigilant to the possibility of this association.

> The patient was a 26-year-old Hispanic man with a history of bipolar disorder who had been stabilized on risperidone 3 mg/day and divalproex sodium 1,500 mg/day. He had been taking these medications at these dosages for more than 1 year. He had no history of trazodone exposure and had no history of vascular disease or other systemic risk factors for priapism. He then developed a 5-day history of persistent erection, dysuria, and urinary incontinence. The erection persisted despite two irrigations of the corpora cavernosa with phenylephrine. He was taken to urological surgery and had a cavernosal glandular shunt and corpora cavernosum–corpus spongiosum shunt performed. Due to the prolonged priapism, he had a 90% risk of permanent erectile dysfunction. Risperidone was discontinued and olanzapine 10 mg at bedtime and paroxetine 20 mg daily were added.

> ◆ **Diagnosis: Axis I—Bipolar Disorder Not Otherwise Specified, 296.80; Adverse Effects of Medication Not Otherwise Specified, 995.2**

Psychiatrists are quite aware of the possibility of priapism in patients prescribed the antidepressant trazodone; indeed, priapism is the major serious side effect (albeit rare) associated with this generally well-tolerated medication. Although again likely rare, priapism has been associated with antipsychotic agents as well. This possibility should be considered in male patients receiving antipsychotic agents who present with priapism, and after medical and/or surgical management of the priapism, alternative psychopharmacological agents should be considered.

References

Davol P, Rukstalis D: Priapism associated with routine use of quetiapine: a case report and review of the literature. Urology 6:880, 2005

Folstein MF, Folstein SE, McHugh PR: "Mini-Mental State": a practical method for grading the cognitive state of patients for the clinician. J Psychiatr Res 12:189–198, 1975

Harrison G, Dilley JS, Loeb L, et al: Priapism and quetiapine: a case report. Psychopharmacol Bull 39:117–119, 2006

Pais VM, Ayvazia PJ: Priapism from quetiapine overdose: first report and proposal of mechanism. Urology 58:462, 2001

Prochaska JO, DiClemente CC: Stages of change in the modification of problem behaviors, in Progress in Behavior Modification, No 28. Edited by Hersen M, Eisler RM, Miller PM. New York, Academic, 1992, pp 184–218

Prochaska JO, DiClemente CC, Norcross JC: In search of how people change: applications to addictive behaviors. Am Psychol 47:1102–1114, 1992

Van der Does AJW, Hinderink EMC, Vloemans AFPM, et al: Burn injuries, psychiatric disorders and length of hospitalization. J Psychosom Res 43:431–435, 1997

13

ORGAN TRANSPLANTATION

Organ transplant cases are among the most interesting and challenging cases in psychosomatic medicine. Involvement in the pretransplant assessment of patients is a critical role for the psychosomatic medicine team and an opportunity for interspecialty collegiality. Patients receiving transplant surgery must commit to lifelong medication compliance and follow-up. The underlying illness leading to the need for transplant (e.g., substance abuse in liver failure) must be concurrently managed. Finally, helping patients deal with the disappointment of organ rejection (which may sadly occur despite the best efforts of medical personnel and patients) is also sometimes necessary.

Kidney Rejection and Depression

The patient was a 26-year-old married, African American male university student. He was admitted to the medical center transplant service for rejection of his transplanted kidney. He had been a very successful track and field athlete, "world class" in the 400-meter sprint, and had been awarded a track and field scholarship to a major university. He was considered a possible prospect for the Olympic Games. Unfortunately, in his first year at the university, he developed an acute streptococcal pharyngitis. Some weeks later, he developed poststreptococcal glomerulonephritis. This illness led to his developing chronic renal failure, which led to his loss of his track and field scholarship, forcing him to leave the university.

Over the next 2 years, he struggled with his progressive renal failure, eventually requiring dialysis. The contrast between his previously highly successful and emotionally gratifying life as a robust and healthy athlete and his later life as a chronically fatigued and dialysis-dependent renal-failure patient was profound. After a period of dialysis, he received a renal transplant operation at age 20.

Although subsequently unable to return to competitive track and field, he was eventually able to return to full-time work and school at a different university. Nonetheless, this was a significantly different and more limited life than he had experienced previously.

Three years later, his girlfriend of several months became pregnant. Although ambivalent about marriage ("because I was never sure she was the right person"), he married her ("it was just the right thing to do"). However, their marriage was stormy. His wife was not able to get along with his family members, resulting in significant distance between him and his family. Notably, his wife was the sister of a National Football League player. His wife would emphasize the athletic and financial success of her brother over the patient's relatively low level of function. Because the patient continued to think of himself as the failed former athlete, the contrast between the patient and his brother-in-law was particularly striking.

Several months prior to his hospital presentation, he began to develop graft rejection. Concurrently, his marriage continued to deteriorate and the couple pursued divorce. He struggled mightily to avoid dialysis, but as it became evident that his renal failure was irreversible, he became depressed with positive neurovegetative signs.

When he was seen in consultation, his affect was dysphoric and restricted. He was nonsuicidal. He was in a stance of negotiation and rationalization. He was begun on a trial of citalopram. Several days after admission, he received a nephrectomy of the failed transplant. Subsequent psychotherapy work focused on assisting him to adjust to his new status as a dialysis patient and instilling a sense of hope for eventual retransplantation. By the end of the hospitalization 10 days after admission, he was more resigned to and accepting of the reality of having to accept dialysis, and he was busily involved in making his discharge and follow-up arrangements. His mood and affect were substantially improved. He was continued on citalopram as an outpatient.

◆ Diagnosis: Axis I—Depressive Disorder Not Otherwise Specified, 311

The contrast between the psychological "high highs" and "low lows" in this patient's life is striking. He had significant and even enviable narcissistic success and gratifying rewards in his time as a track and field star. Then, suddenly, he was felled by a disabling illness. He was quite in touch with the sense of loss this represented. He struggled for years with illness, eventually capitulating to dialysis, then welcoming a renal transplant. He was subsequently profoundly disappointed that his horizons would be forever limited, despite the receipt of a new kidney. The recurrence of his renal failure and realization of the likely need for resumption of dialysis was a significant narcissistic injury associated with an understandable onset of depressive symptoms.

The contrast between his prior success in athletics, his later loss of athletic identity, and the painful and regular reminder of this loss whenever he was confronted with his athletically successful brother-in-law was most painful for him. He told the psychiatrist, "I realize how unlikely it is to make it in professional sports. There are only about 5,000 jobs. Yet I was so close." In the psychotherapy approach to this patient, his sense of self-efficacy was mobilized as a method to encourage him to adjust and to accept dialysis as a bridge to an eventual retransplantation.

Paranoia, Renal Transplantation, and Noncompliance

The patient was a 47-year-old divorced Central American man who spoke little English. He had received a renal transplant 7 years previously due to diabetic kidney disease, which had rendered him dialysis dependent. Notably, he had had no history of psychiatric illness or substance abuse at the time, and there were no behavioral concerns about his ability to function compliantly as a renal transplant patient. He received his transplant uneventfully and was seen regularly in outpatient clinic for follow-up for several years.

However, he later presented acutely to the medical center with threatened kidney rejection and altered mental status, with a high white blood cell count consistent with infection and possible sepsis. He was admitted to the transplant surgery service for medical management. A family member had indicated to the transplant service that the patient had been "behaving strangely" for some time prior to admission, and there was concern that he had been noncompliant with his antirejection medications. On initial clinical interview, he was obviously confused and disoriented and could not answer questions appropriately. A psychosomatic medicine consultation was called to "evaluate mental status changes."

When he was seen for evaluation, a far more intriguing picture quickly emerged. He was interviewed each time with a Spanish-speaking nurse or physician to facilitate communication. On initial interview, he told the team that, yes, indeed he had not taken his antirejection medications for "at least 2 months...because they weren't safe...they were going to give me an infection." When asked to elaborate on this concern, he explained that the "contamination" in his home had allowed "bacteria to leak in through the cracks in the walls." The "bacteria" had subsequently found their way into the bottles containing his antirejection medications and had "filled them with pus." As such, he could not ingest "pills full of pus." Unfortunately, he had not told any of his physicians of this predicament and had grown increasingly ill until his family members finally brought him to the hospital.

He was treated with aripiprazole 15 mg daily. Over several days, his delusion about his antirejection medications abated significantly. Although early in the hospitalization he had refused them (causing understandably great concern among the transplant surgery team physicians), he later took them cooperatively. However, he continued to maintain that his home was "contaminated with bacteria" and other unspecified but threatening materials. Because his residual delusions were felt to represent an impediment to safe self-care (especially in light of his need for lifelong immunosuppression), he was sent to an inpatient psychiatric unit for consolidation of his antipsychotic treatment once his systemic medical condition was stabilized.

♦ Diagnosis: Axis I—Psychotic Disorder Not Otherwise Specified, 298.9

Psychotic illness, always a potential threat to the patient's integrity, takes on a special urgency in the chronically ill patient for whom daily medication compliance is an imperative. Rarely is this more clearly illustrated than in organ transplant patients. Indeed, psychotic illness is often regarded as either a relative contraindication to transplant surgery or at least a matter of significant clinical concern preoperatively.

Curious in this man's case was the fact that the psychotic illness developed several years postoperatively. The theme of "bacteria" contaminating first his home and then later his medications was most impressive. Once the medications were "contaminated" in this way, routine medication compliance became impossible for him. This quickly became unsustainable, with hospitalization resulting. Prompt evaluation of his psychotic illness and prompt institution of antipsychotic medication was associated with an improvement in his delusions to the point at which medication compliance could be resumed.

Given this man's need for indefinite treatment with antirejection medications, maintenance antipsychotic therapy needs to be strongly considered. Psychosomatic medicine psychiatrists confronting the noncompliant posttransplant patient (a cohort of patients that induce considerable countertransference feelings in transplant clinicians, who make the expectation of posttransplant compliance an imperative) should consider the possibility of "psychotic noncompliance" in cases such as this one and offer appropriate antipsychotic therapy.

New-Onset Seizure in a Transplant Patient: Surreptitious Benzodiazepine Withdrawal, Bupropion Side Effect, or Both?

Organ transplantation patients are commonly complex in terms of medical and surgical morbidity, pharmacological treatment, and psychiatric history. Often these patients are encountered in a setting of acute illness when previous interventions have been inadequate. Because of the complexity of such cases, it is often difficult to be certain how to attribute unexpected and unfortunate clinical events. These variables are additive to the often long struggles these patients have had in dealing with their chronic illness, their dependency on medical and surgical interventions, and their frequent disease progression despite the most well-intended clinical interventions.

> The patient was a 52-year-old married white man. He had had chronic kidney disease since childhood and had already had one renal transplant eventually followed by graft failure. Subsequently, he received a second renal transplant. Unfortunately, the second renal allograft also failed to function, and he became once again dialysis dependent. He was admitted to the medical center for surgical exploration of the failed allograft, which had become the cause of complications. He was admitted for the procedure, which was successful without any intraoperative or postoperative complications. Three days postoperatively, a psychosomatic medicine consultation was called because of a "history of depression." Notably, his psychiatric history had not been of sufficient concern preoperatively to generate a clinic transplant evaluation before the admission.
>
> When seen for formal consultation, he revealed a long psychiatric history of recurrent episodes of recurrent depression, dating to his early adult years. He had been treated with multiple selective serotonin reuptake inhibitors (SSRIs), with generally favorable results. He had not been taking antidepressants immediately prior to the admission. On examination, he was mildly dysphoric, nonsuicidal, and

nonpsychotic. His cognitive status was unremarkable, with a Mini-Mental State Examination (MMSE; Folstein et al. 1975) score of 28. Although obviously disappointed at the failure of his second renal allograft, he was nonsuicidal and was willing to commit to follow-up psychiatric treatment for his recurrent depression. His history was negative for eating disorder or seizure disorder. Because he had had equivocal response to SSRIs historically, he was started on bupropion extended release 150 mg every morning and quetiapine 25 mg at bedtime. When he was seen again the next day, his condition was unchanged.

Later that evening, he received opioid pain medication. When seen for follow-up the next morning, he had deteriorated significantly. His renal function was noted to have declined. He now had a variable level of consciousness and gross confusion. His MMSE score had deteriorated to 6. He was now diagnosed with delirium, which was initially related to worse renal function and the use of opioids. When seen later that day, he was somnolent and minimally arousable. His MMSE score was now 0. It was recommended to hold opioids and to recheck mental status after dialysis, which was scheduled for later that day.

The next morning, after a dialysis treatment, he was more alert but his cognitive status was still impaired, with an MMSE score of 10. Quetiapine was now held. The next morning, he exhibited notable and new motor agitation, hypertension, and tachycardia. He was also more confused. Later that day, he was observed to have some tonic-clonic seizure activity and subsequent minimal responsiveness. Following the seizure activity, lorazepam was started. At this point, additional data (previously unavailable) were obtained; notably, he had been on diazepam (Valium) and temazepam (Restoril) before the admission (he had denied having used benzodiazepines when seen for initial consultation). In light of the clinical changes and the history of benzodiazepine exposure, benzodiazepine withdrawal was now suspected. Because of the seizure activity, bupropion and quetiapine were now held.

For airway protection, he was intubated and transferred to the intensive care unit. An electroencephalogram was obtained and revealed bilateral diffuse slowing consistent with delirium. Notably, no seizure focus was identified. With continued care in the intensive care unit and use of lorazepam, his vital signs renormalized and his agitation resolved. When interviewed 4 days later (having been transferred out of intensive care), he felt well. He had no memory of the period of his seizure activity or his stay in the intensive care unit. When confronted about benzodiazepine use, he now confirmed that he had been using diazepam and temazepam chronically preadmission "to get to sleep." He said that he "was not aware that Valium and Restoril were addictive medications." His cognitive status had improved substantially, with an MMSE score of 25. Sertraline 50 mg every morning was started, and plans for outpatient psychiatry follow-up were made.

◆ **Diagnosis: Axis I—Major Depressive Disorder, Recurrent, Moderate, 296.32; Sedative, Hypnotic, or Anxiolytic Dependence, 304.10; Sedative, Hypnotic, or Anxiolytic Withdrawal, 292.0; Delirium, 293.0**

This man's history was notable for his having been a long-term survivor of childhood renal disease and having received two renal transplants. Despite the best efforts of all involved, the second renal transplant had failed, leading to his admission. Surely, his risk of recurrent depression in the context of chronic renal disease is understandably high. When initially encountered in the hospital, given his long depression history and the need for reinstitution of antidepressant treatment, the decision to begin bupropion was appropriate. The initial consultant dutifully obtained a history of no seizures before bupropion was started.

Unfortunately, the history of chronic use of benzodiazepines was not initially known. The patient had fully detailed his history of treatment with several different antidepressants but had withheld the history of benzodiazepine use. Five days after admission (and 2 days after starting bupropion) he developed altered mental status and subsequently suffered a seizure. He had autonomic instability that was responsive to a short course of lorazepam, and he promptly cleared. Because the seizure occurred within a few days of starting bupropion, which has a well-known (if slight) associated risk of seizures, bupropion was necessarily held. Although it would be very problematic (in case of another seizure) to resume bupropion in a patient who had had a seizure within 1 week of having started it, one must wonder if in fact the two clinical events were related at all.

It is possible (if not likely) that the seizure was solely the consequence of benzodiazepine withdrawal, because the time course of onset of symptoms was classic. Clinicians admitting patients (especially those with complicated histories) should be vigilant for the (possibly surreptitious) use of benzodiazepines. Admitting physicians may consider routinely obtaining toxicology screens for hospital admissions to identify such cases; this seems especially reasonable when patients are admitted specifically for planned surgical procedures. One wonders how many cases of "straightforward postoperative delirium" may (in part) be "sedative, hypnotic, or anxiolytic withdrawal delirium."

Recurrent Major Depression and Altruistic Renal Donation

Organ transplantation services are often skeptical of the motivation of a volunteer kidney donor who voluntarily steps forward to donate to an unknown other as a purely altruistic act. Transplant centers may routinely request psychosomatic medicine consultation on such patients before allowing them to donate. One of the authors had a striking case of a physician who volunteered to donate. In addition to the fascinating psychodynamic aspects of this case, there was a serious recurrent mood disorder to assess.

> The patient was a 60-year-old married white male physician. He presented to the transplant service with the desire to be a renal donor. When seen in consultation, he presented in a controlled and matter-of-fact manner. He had been married for 26 years and had one stepdaughter and two daughters. He was very close to his stepdaughter, who tragically had recently been widowed. The patient's deceased stepson-in-law, the spouse of this woman, had had a complicated and lingering battle with juvenile-onset insulin-dependent diabetes mellitus. He had been a kidney-pancreas transplant recipient who initially responded well to the transplant, only to die later of a myocardial infarction. The patient's experience of grief over this family member's death crystallized his desire to donate a kidney as an altruistic act.
>
> The patient was a primary care physician who had recently semi-retired. He explained that now that he was semi-retired, he wanted to donate a kidney because it was "time to perform a generous act." Notably, he had a long-standing participation in medical missionary work overseas. He denied any coercive or financial pressures to donate or any family resistance to his desire to be an organ donor.
>
> Such volunteer altruistic or unrelated donor offers are relatively rare, and it was even rarer for a still-practicing physician to offer to donate an organ. Complicating the case was his quite remarkable history of recurrent major depression, about which he was quite "up front" and open to discussion. He had a strong family history of

depression on his mother's side. His maternal grandfather had had depression, as had his mother and her four sisters (the patient's aunts), two of whom died of self-inflicted gunshot wounds. He also had two brothers with depression.

The patient had had five episodes of major depression with neurovegetative signs including recurrent suicidal ideation. The first depressive episode was at age 21 when he was a university student. Despite significant mood symptoms at the time, including weight loss and suicidal ideation, he was not medicated for this episode. He recovered spontaneously after several months.

The second episode of major depression was in his mid-20s, as a medical student. His symptoms were similar to those of the initial episode. He briefly attended psychotherapy, but again was not medicated. The symptoms again resolved spontaneously after several months. The third episode was at age 40, while he served as senior administrator at his hospital. Again, he did not receive medication, and his depression resolved in several months. The fourth episode was at age 44. He was treated with fluoxetine, to which he had a prompt and robust response.

The fifth episode, the most serious one, was at age 50. He had had a 45-pound weight loss and persistent suicidal ideation and had attempted suicide by intentionally causing a single-vehicle motor vehicle accident. He attended 1 month of partial hospitalization and was tried on several medication combinations. He was eventually stabilized on venlafaxine (extended release, 75 mg daily), bupropion (sustained release, 150 mg daily), and trazodone (50 mg daily at bedtime). At the time of the preoperative evaluation, he was stable and compliant with medications. He readily accepted the need for medications and considered himself committed to lifelong treatment.

He was able to discuss his interest in renal donation in a calm and matter-of-fact manner. His sense of altruism, based on his professional career, his voluntary overseas medical missionary service, and his interest in donating a kidney to an anonymous stranger, was striking and notable. His mood disorder was well treated, and he had no current depressive symptoms. He was cleared for renal donor status.

◆ **Diagnosis: Axis I—Major Depressive Disorder, Recurrent, in Remission, 296.36**

The psychosomatic medicine physician's role in this case, as a consultant to the renal transplant program, was twofold. The paradox is that the patient who comes forward spontaneously to offer to be a renal donor, obviously a profoundly generous act, requires psychiatric clearance for the donation. Perhaps others are concerned that the donor is seeking to alleviate excess (if somewhat nonspecified) guilt by the single act of organ donation, or perhaps such an out-of-the-ordinary act of generosity seems so far beyond normative behavior (recall the worldwide shortage of transplantable organs, largely attributable to the unwillingness of families to allow for organ donation even after the death of a loved one) that there is inherent suspicion of someone who would present in such a context.

Obviously, the possibility exists that someone may volunteer to be an "altruistic" donor in the context of depression-driven excess guilt, or perhaps out a sense of grandiosity in untreated bipolar disorder, or even as part of a delusional belief system in a psychotic disorder. If so, these psychiatric illnesses could be discovered in a diagnostic interview. It is also possible that some "apparent" altruistic donors are in a surreptitious way being influenced by perverse incentives such as coercive (if secret) financial compensation offers. Such motivation may be extremely hard to discern in interview, especially if the donor is motivated to continue to maintain secrecy.

In this man's case, the fact that he was a physician and had suffered the loss of a family member who had himself been a kidney transplant recipient added a bit of intrigue. Extending the usual "other-centeredness" one finds desirable in a physician colleague (and, indeed, aspires to oneself), this man had gone "beyond" normative physician behavior by dint of his many overseas travels to assist others by the provision of medical services. Notably, he recounted these overseas travels in a manner that did not bring attention to his efforts; in fact, he was quite modest about his motivation, saying that overseas medical missionary work was merely something he felt compelled to do, not that he particularly sought external affirmation. Although he did not directly relate the personal need to donate a kidney to somehow indirectly compensating for the tragic loss of his stepson-in-law by helping another renal failure patient, no doubt consciousness of this loss played a role in affirming his motivation.

Beyond these considerations, clearly significant in their own right and on their own quite adequate to make this a memorable case, was the patient's own history of recurrent major depression. He recounted his mood disorder history (including the significant family history) in a notably direct way. He was completely accepting of his psychiatric history and readily agreed to the need for indefinite psychopharmacological and psychiatric care, and he credited his ongoing relationship with his psychiatrist with maintaining his ability to function highly as a senior physician.

This man's story was quite inspirational. Having worked a long and productive career despite the obvious personal setbacks due to his recurrent depression, he was under no external obligation to offer himself as a renal donor. Notable was his calm, reasoned, and matter-of-fact manner about this issue. This was a remarkably generous act in a generous life and an inspirational reminder of seeking out the most that one can do for others.

Posttransplant Catatonia and Psychosis

Case 1

A 50-year-old Filipino man with chronic hepatitis C was treated with a course of interferon and ribavirin therapy; however, despite the interferon therapy, he progressed to liver failure and transplant listing. Notably, he had no prior psychiatric history other than a brief period of intravenous drug use in his youth (the likely cause of his hepatitis C exposure) and tolerated his (ultimately noncurative) course of interferon without psychiatric complications. He had been living in the United States for more than 20 years, although he maintained a strong Filipino cultural identity. He had been employed in manufacturing before progressive disability from liver failure required him to stop working. In the process of transplant evaluation, no psychosocial contraindications to transplantation were noted, and his candidacy proceeded without difficulty.

When he was called to the medical center for his liver transplant operation, there were no undue psychiatric concerns. He received the liver of a young male trauma victim. There were no operative complications. He did not experience postoperative delirium. However, several days postoperatively, his behavior changed radically. Normally a friendly and engaging man, he became progressively less verbal to the point of mutism. Concurrently, he would keep his incentive spirometer clenched tightly in his mouth while twisting the rest of the device in a ritualistic fashion. He remained alert and otherwise cooperative, without agitation. He would protest if a staff member attempted to remove the spirometer from his mouth.

On psychosomatic medicine consultation, he was found to be alert and nonverbal. He continued to hold the spirometer clenched in his mouth and was apparently purposelessly twisting it in his hands. Due to his nonverbal state, the balance of the psychiatric examination could not be completed. He was diagnosed with acute catatonia and treated with lorazepam 1 mg orally every 6 hours. Within 24 hours, he released the spirometer from his mouth and began to speak. He then told the psychosomatic medicine team that he was holding the spirometer in his mouth because he had been told that if he did not perform adequate spirometry exercises postoperatively, he would "lose the new liver." In addition, he was experiencing paranoid ideation that nonspecified "government agents" would come into his room and "take the new liver" because he was "unworthy of having the transplant." Furthermore, he had somehow learned that the donor was a young adult trauma patient, and the fact that his transplant was made possible by the tragic death of another man was associated with significant guilt for him.

Because he was no longer catatonic, lorazepam was then discontinued. Due to the now evident psychotic symptoms, he was started on quetiapine and followed closely with supportive psychotherapy. Over a period of several days, his paranoia resolved and his mood improved. He was able to return home after several more days in the hospital. He was seen in clinical follow-up over the next 18 months (during which time quetiapine was tapered and discontinued) with no recurrence of either catatonia or psychotic symptoms.

◆ **Diagnosis: Axis I—Catatonic Disorder Due to a General Medical Condition, 293.89; Brief Psychotic Disorder, 298.8**

This fascinating case reminds the psychosomatic medicine psychiatrist to have an observant eye for catatonia with any acute presentation of dramatically changed mental status and be willing to quickly initiate an empirical trial of lorazepam (Fink and Taylor 2001; Taylor and Fink 2003). In this case, the catatonic behavior quickly improved, only to reveal the presence of a profound (yet of remarkably brief duration) delusional belief system. The paranoid delusions were thematically related to psychiatric aspects of the transplant, including his guilt that another patient had to die to make his transplant possible, a type of survivor guilt.

Prompt recognition of the "uncovered" delusional symptoms led to a trial of quetiapine, which was associated with prompt improvement in the psychotic symptoms. It is possible that this case represented postoperative delirium with a catatonic and paranoid presentation; indeed, this cannot be ruled out completely. The fact that there was a strong dynamic theme of his not having been worthy of the transplant, a sense of guilt that another man's death had served to provide the needed liver, and delusional misunderstanding of his postoperative recovery instructions are all consistent with a psychodynamic explanation of some of his symptoms. Psychosomatic medicine physicians need to be alert to the possibility of the presentation of catatonic behavior, whether this is attributed to a discrete catatonic episode or as a regressed form of delirium.

Case 2

The patient was a 52-year-old Hispanic man who spoke only Spanish. He had no history of psychiatric illness beyond his substance abuse, which was now in remission. He had a history of hepatitis B and cirrhosis, for which he had received a liver transplant 5 years earlier. He initially did well after his transplant, but over the interceding years, he eventually developed recurrence of cirrhosis in his transplanted liver. By the time he presented to the medical center for a second liver transplant, he was experiencing hepatorenal syndrome, which necessitated a combined liver and kidney transplant.

His operation went well, and postoperatively, he quickly established improved liver and kidney function. However, within a few days of his operation, he began to voice paranoid delusions. He cried out that the nurses in the intensive care unit were "trying to kill me by choking me" and that the medical staff "wanted to tear me apart." Concurrently with these new paranoid delusions, he developed motor agitation and refused all medications (including his immunosuppressants), fearful that they were "poison." Because of a new onset of psychosis, a psychosomatic medicine consultation was ordered.

However, before the team was able to evaluate the patient several hours later, his behavior deteriorated and regressed markedly. He had previously been spontaneously verbal about his paranoid delusions, but he now had no coherent spontaneous speech. He had a vacant, "distant" gaze and did not make eye contact. He was unable to perform any formal cognitive examination items and did not respond to routine questions about suicidality, homicidality, or psychosis. He did not appear to recognize his wife, who was visiting at the bedside. She was able (through an interpreter) to tell the team that he had never exhibited this kind of regressed behavior before and that he had not had any behavioral problems following his initial liver transplant operation. Notably, he was no longer voicing the paranoid delusions so prominent only a few hours earlier. His only intelligible verbal responses were notable echolalia, where he would repeat the English statements of the examiners (despite being able to speak only a few English words). He was fully alert and did not exhibit motor agitation, although he demonstrated notable posturing (strongly clutching the bed sheets with both hands).

He was diagnosed with catatonia. Because of the antecedent psychotic symptoms, he was treated concurrently with lorazepam 1 mg every 6 hours for the catatonia and olanzapine 5 mg every 12 hours for the paranoid delusions. Within 48 hours, his catatonic behavior had resolved. He was now appropriately interactive, responded with appropriate verbal responses, and had no further posturing. He had no further paranoid delusions and had no suicidal or homicidal ideation. His MMSE score was 23. Lorazepam was tapered and discontinued. He was shortly thereafter transferred from intensive care to the ward for further observation; olanzapine was decreased to 5 mg at bedtime.

Unfortunately, on his first evening on the hospital ward, there was a fire drill on his nursing unit. Frightened by the commotion and activity, and not understanding that this was merely a training exercise, he had a brief recurrence of his paranoia. He became agitated and needed an extra dose of olanzapine. Upon interview the next morning, his cognitive testing was stable, and he was able to tell us of the fear that he was "trapped" in his hospital room the night before. Out of concern for residual paranoid ideation (although it is likely the environmental stimulus of the fire drill may have been responsible for his recurrence), his olanzapine was increased to 5 mg every 12 hours. For the next several days of hospitalization, he had no further paranoia and no recurrence of catatonia. He was able (through an interpreter) to discuss his having been paranoid, but he had no memory of his brief period of catatonia. He was discharged in stable condition on olanzapine with a slow taper schedule over 2 weeks, with instructions to seek emergent care for any recurrence of mental status changes.

◆ **Diagnosis: Axis I—Catatonic Disorder Due to a General Medical Condition, 293.89; Brief Psychotic Disorder, 298.8**

This case has some similarities to the previous one. In each case, the patient had no history of psychosis or catatonia until the postoperative period. In each case, there was a brief period of persecutory delusions (with a medical/surgical theme) preceding the deterioration into catatonia, with largely nonverbal behavior, posturing, and in the second case, echolalia. Because of the antecedent psychosis symptoms followed by catatonia, the treatment chosen was lorazepam for the catatonic component and an antipsychotic for the paranoid component. In the second case, the catatonia quickly resolved, but the paranoid delusions briefly returned during the hospitalization. Adjustment of the antipsychotic medication was associated with prompt improvement. Because there is little literature to guide the clinician on the indefinite management of these patients, we chose to maintain the antipsychotic agent briefly following discharge, emphasizing the need for clinical follow-up in case of recurrence.

Social Phobia, Alcohol Dependence, and Liver Transplantation

Substance dependence is, of course, common in patients receiving hepatic transplantation. Thus, psychosomatic medicine services are intimately involved with this patient population. Often, the pretransplantation evaluation leads to a diagnosis of psychiatric comorbidity that may be implicated in the genesis of the substance abuse. Treatment of these comorbid conditions may be necessary to help maintain preoperative sobriety and recovery and posttransplant compliance with immunosuppressant medications. Because of the timing of presentation of various psychiatric syndromes, however, initial evaluation may be focused on the management of postoperative delirium, with discovery and management of comorbid conditions possible after initial management of delirium.

> The patient was a 50-year-old married white woman. She had had no formal psychiatric history aside from the gradual development of alcohol dependence. As a result, she developed cirrhosis and required a transplant operation. Fortunately for her transplant candidacy, she was otherwise a high-functioning patient with excellent sources of social support for the peri- and posttransplant period. She was able to commit to sobriety and attended Alcoholics Anonymous meetings as required by the transplantation service, and she was listed for the transplant operation.
>
> When an organ became available, she was admitted and underwent a successful liver transplantation. Her new liver functioned well without any evidence of rejection. However, several days postoperatively, she developed an episode of delirium. She acutely

developed paranoid ideations about the medical center "not being safe" and that medical center staff were "threatening" her with unspecified harm. She also experienced visual and auditory hallucinations of various people in her hospital room; at times she was observed in active conversation as if with these hallucinations. She was successfully treated with olanzapine 5 mg orally at bedtime; her psychotic symptoms quickly cleared, and by discharge time she was doing well, with normal cognitive status.

She was continued on olanzapine after discharge and was seen in psychosomatic medicine clinical follow-up approximately 6 weeks later. At that point, she felt well, without any recurrence of the psychotic symptoms that she had experienced during her episode of delirium. She was able to remember "fragments" of symptoms that had occurred during her delirium episode, but she was not unduly troubled by these and was readily able to understand them as a transient experience that was not expected to recur. She remained committed to continued Alcoholics Anonymous attendance and a program of recovery/sobriety. She regarded her transplant as a "new opportunity" in life, and for this she was profoundly grateful.

During this follow-up visit, she was able to now describe a 20-year history of tonic baseline anxiety that increased to panic level in certain social situations involving public scrutiny by other people. Her father and daughter had the same behavioral condition; her daughter had been in psychiatric treatment and was now doing better. She was now able to connect how her previous pattern of alcohol use had been primarily motivated by the need for an anxiolytic to tolerate forced social situations, which would have been extremely difficult for her otherwise. This pattern had escalated to her previous pattern of alcohol dependence.

Because she was now several weeks past her delirium episode, olanzapine was discontinued. She was started on citalopram 20 mg every morning and alprazolam 0.25 mg every 8 hours as needed for severe anxiety. Several days later, she telephoned to say that the citalopram was associated with a feeling of increased anxiety and feeling unpleasantly "wired." Citalopram was then discontinued and mirtazapine 15 mg at bedtime was started. This medication was associated immediately with better sleep and appetite, much less baseline and socially cued anxiety, and no need to use alprazolam.

◆ **Diagnosis: Axis I—Delirium (in Remission), 293.0; Alcohol Dependence (in Remission), 303.90; Generalized Anxiety Disorder, 300.02; Social Phobia, 300.23**

This pattern of substance dependence (primarily alcohol and sed-atives/hypnotics) may be seen in social phobia patients who discover the effect of sedatives on their social anxiety. In this patient's case, this pattern escalated to the point of needing liver transplantation. Her immediate postoperative period was characterized by a delirium with notable psychotic features. This was managed, and once she was no longer delirious, her long-standing pattern of social anxiety lead-ing to alcohol dependence could be assessed and treated. Psychoso-matic medicine physicians may occasionally see this pattern of substance use in their liver transplant patients; conventional inter-ventions for social phobia are indicated to optimize patient function.

Panic Disorder, Alcohol Dependence, and Liver Failure

In transplant psychiatry work, the more usual case may be a patient with a primary substance dependence disorder (most commonly al-cohol), which has resulted in the liver disease and liver failure. Rou-tinely, transplant surgery teams expect sobriety for a convincing pe-riod of time, acceptance of addiction and need for treatment, a stable social environment, and compliance with pretransplant clinical ser-vices before a liver transplant surgery is offered. The transplant psy-chiatrist's role in such cases includes evaluation and management of additional psychopathology, evaluation and monitoring of the cog-nitive status (especially in patients with risk of episodes of hepatic en-cephalopathy), and affirmation of the sobriety plan. Occasionally, a patient will present in whom a long-standing and undertreated psy-chiatric disorder is the primary problem, with compensatory sub-stance dependence in the form of "self-medication" resulting in liver failure and the need for transplant surgery. However, sometimes the nature of the premorbid psychiatric illness itself (if not appropriately managed) makes the patient unable to comply with the usual care ex-pectations of the transplant surgery service, putting the patient at risk of being labeled noncompliant and denied the very transplant he or she needs for survival.

The patient was a 51-year-old, twice-divorced white woman who was on disability due to liver disease. She had been admitted to a community hospital 5 years before with the acute onset of liver failure. At that time, she had been escalating her alcohol use to a typical daily use of "24 beers." When confronted about her liver disease, she immediately discontinued her alcohol use but was unable to attend Alcoholics Anonymous "because I am afraid to speak in public and participate in groups." She had several episodes of hepatic encephalopathy over the next several years and was referred to the medical center for evaluation for liver transplantation. When she appeared (reluctantly) at the transplant center, she presented in an anxious, fearful, and depressed manner. On initial review by the transplant team, concern was raised over her "lack of insight into her alcoholism" and "resistance" to attending Alcoholics Anonymous as putting her at risk for noncompliance. Because of these concerns, an outpatient psychosomatic medicine consultation was arranged.

When she presented for her outpatient evaluation, a far more complex picture emerged. The patient described having been raised by an "always depressed and often physically and verbally abusive" mother. In addition, both of her parents and three of her siblings were alcoholics who never participated in recovery activities or achieved sobriety. She was largely estranged from her family members as a result. She developed a lifelong pattern of social avoidance, fearfulness at attending events in public, and beginning in her 20s, recurrent spontaneous panic attacks with increasingly agoraphobic behavior. She had had the panic symptoms for many months before approaching her primary care physician for initial treatment. She was treated with alprazolam for a period of several years, during which time her panic symptoms improved. Her pattern of social avoidance persisted. After several years of decreased panic attacks, her alprazolam was discontinued.

Not surprisingly, without the alprazolam, her panic disorder symptoms recurred over time. However, this time she did not seek medical attention. She began to self-medicate with alcohol, about which she had considerable shame and guilt but thought that she "couldn't help it." Her pattern of alcohol dependence accelerated until she was regularly drinking 24 beers per day. She had been married and divorced twice during this period. After her hospitalization for liver failure, she was able to stop drinking alcohol but did not seek psychiatric care for her underlying panic disorder. She had attempted to attend Alcoholics Anonymous on a few occasions but became very fearful in the meetings and was never able to introduce herself or to tell her story in a meeting. Eventually, she ceased even trying to attend meetings. She became increasingly reclusive, eventually becoming unable to work and having minimal social contacts. She felt very guilty over becoming an alcoholic and having alcoholic liver disease. She became increasingly depressed, with poor sleep and appetite, but was never suicidal. She had not previously sought treatment for her mood disorder.

Examination revealed an anxious, tearful, dysphoric middle-aged woman who appeared much older than her stated age. She was non-suicidal and nonpsychotic but clearly ashamed of her alcoholism and fearful that the transplant team saw her as "just an alcoholic." She said that she did not enjoy the taste of alcohol and did not like the feeling of intoxication, but that she had only used alcohol to self-medicate otherwise paralyzing anxiety. Her MMSE score was 28. The formulation of avoidant personality disorder, panic disorder, major depression, and alcohol dependence was presented in depth, and she readily appreciated how this formulation described her experience accurately. Most importantly, the personality disorder and panic disorder were presented as the "primary" clinical problem and the alcohol dependence as "secondary." It was further explained how it was quite difficult (if not impossible) to expect a patient with avoidant personality disorder and untreated panic disorder to somehow be able to tolerate the "maximum phobic stimulus" of required attendance and active participation in Alcoholics Anonymous, a conclusion that the patient embraced with considerable and palpable relief. She was treated with mirtazapine 15 mg at bedtime and lorazepam 0.5 mg every 6 hours as needed for panic attacks.

When seen in follow-up 4 weeks later, she reported that her sleep was "the best I have had in years." Her mood was much better and more hopeful; her affect was notably bright and not at all anxious. She now had only infrequent episodes of panic-level anxiety; these episodes responded promptly to the dose of lorazepam. On other episodes of panic, she was able to tolerate the anxiety knowing it would pass and said that "just having it [lorazepam] available was reassuring." With her mood and anxiety symptoms finally improved, she was able (wistfully) to observe that she wished she had gotten proper treatment long ago so as to have avoided her alcoholic liver disease. However, she had an increased sense of self-confidence to now pursue the workup for liver transplantation. The psychosomatic medicine psychiatrist communicated to the transplant surgery team that with her clinical recovery and commitment to further treatment, this patient was now an acceptable candidate for liver transplant surgery.

◆ **Diagnosis: Axis I—Panic Disorder With Agoraphobia, 300.21; Major Depressive Disorder, Single Episode, Moderate, 296.22; Alcohol Dependence (in Remission), 303.90; Delirium (in Remission), 293.0; Axis II—Avoidant Personality Disorder, 301.82**

This patient's pattern of social avoidance and shyness with reclusive behavior may be dynamically attributed to having been raised in a chaotic home with multiple substance abusers. Her later development of panic disorder is hardly surprising; the tragic choice of alcohol as a self-medication for anxiolysis led to eventual liver failure and the need for transplant. The "usual and routine" expectations of the transplant service for regular and committed active attendance at Alcoholics Anonymous meetings as a minimal condition for transplant candidacy presented her with an intolerable dilemma. To attend and make witness at Alcoholics Anonymous meetings (a challenge for many patients, to be sure) is an overwhelming phobic stimulus for the unfortunate patient with (untreated) panic disorder and avoidant personality disorder. Her later development of depression is understandable in light of her clinical and social deterioration. Comprehensive psychopharmacological and psychotherapeutic intervention and courageous self-examination by the patient resulted in the possibility of saving her liver transplant candidacy and allowing her to receive life-enhancing treatment.

References

Fink M, Taylor MA: The many varieties of catatonia. Eur Arch Psychiatry Clin Neurosci 251(suppl):1/8–1/13, 2001

Folstein MF, Folstein SE, McHugh PR: "Mini-Mental State": a practical method for grading the cognitive state of patients for the clinician. J Psychiatr Res 12:189–198, 1975

Taylor MA, Fink M: Catatonia in psychiatric classification: a home of its own. Am J Psychiatry 160:1233–1242, 2003

14

NEUROLOGY AND NEUROSURGERY

Neurology, neurosurgery, and psychiatry, as three "brain special-ties," share a common interest in overlapping subject matter. There-fore, neurological and neurosurgical illnesses are inherently interesting to psychosomatic medicine psychiatrists. Beyond that, it is understandable that neurological and neurosurgical illnesses are associated with a significant risk of psychiatric symptoms. The chal-lenge to psychosomatic medicine psychiatrists in such cases is often related to modifying the clinical interview to communicate with pa-tients with significant cognitive impairment. In addition, many neu-rological and neurosurgical illnesses are associated with grim prognoses for functional status or survival, so an ability to engage in frank discussions about existential matters is often necessary.

Frontal Dementia in Wilson Disease

The patient was a 48-year-old man with known Wilson disease, first diagnosed when he was in his 20s. He had been intermittently com-pliant with penicillamine therapy and a low-copper diet over the years and had signs of diffuse neurological dysfunction on examina-tion. He was referred by his neurologist for psychiatry evaluation for mood and memory complaints.

The patient revealed that he had had neuropsychological testing nearly 10 years earlier. He said that he was "unimpressed by the rel-evance of the results" to his day-to-day function then, although the report showed that he already had at that time "markedly impaired executive functions, including initiation and mental flexibility, sug-gestive of a process involving frontal and subcortical circuits."

An environmental engineer, he now said "I feel my performance has declined at work. I think I'm just burnt out." He noted particular difficulties with concentration that worsened when his perceived stress level rose. He also said that he had run up bills of many hundreds of dollars on his cell phone several months in a row, and he had "a hard time understanding how that could have happened."

The patient said he wanted the psychiatrist to weigh the perspectives of people close to him. He asked him to call his business partner of 22 years, who described the patient as "very intelligent but recently quite forgetful, with indecisiveness and trouble analyzing a set of facts like he used to." On occasion, particularly when a project was not going well, he had lashed out verbally against coworkers. According to the partner, "It seems like he has had mood swings that come out of the blue and go away as quickly."

Although admitting that they had had marital problems for more than a decade, the patient's wife said that she had seen a marked increase in the insensitivity of the comments he made about her over the past couple of years, stating "He shows me no compassion." In particular, she said he would make remarks she perceived as hateful about her weight or her makeup. She said "He will tell me I look like a fat cow without any expression on his face or in his voice at all!" Furthermore, she had become concerned about his tendency to come home from work and take up residence in his recliner for the evening, watching whatever happened to be on, apparently indifferent to the content: "All he does is sit there staring at the television, doing absolutely nothing. It's just not like him!"

She reported that his behavior had been inappropriate in situations involving alcohol and sex. He recently provided his 16-year-old son and several friends with a case of beer and a fifth of vodka for a school-night party. "What's the problem?" he asked. "I'd rather they get trashed at home than on the streets." He had also attempted to get his 23-year-old daughter to discuss the intimate details of her lovemaking with her boyfriend.

◆ **Diagnosis: Axis I—Dementia Due to a General Medical Condition, With Behavioral Disturbance, 294.11**

This case represents one of the classic frontal-subcortical dementias with three symptom groups: dysexecutive, disinhibition, and apathetic (Bonelli and Cummings 2008; Duffy and Campbell 1994). These are referred to as the three regional prefrontal syndromes and are each associated with dysfunction of separate areas of the prefrontal regions. Because the clinical presentation represents aspects of all three areas of impairment, the clinician should consider this diagnosis and formulation as a parsimonious way to explain a complex presentation. As with many dementia syndromes, the other behavioral disturbances as illustrated in this case are often far more socially disruptive to the patient's function than the cognitive impairment per se.

Parkinson's Disease, Dementia, Delirium, and Polypharmacy Risks

The patient was a frail 89-year-old woman with mild dementia, possible early Parkinson's disease, and moderate hearing and visual loss. After the assisted living center in which she had been living determined that she needed more care than it could provide, her daughter and son-in-law took her into their home rather than permitting her to be sent to a nursing home. For the previous 2 years they had provided exemplary care, and she was comfortable and happy in their home.

However, they noticed that when both of them were away at the same time, particularly at night, she became restive and frightened, calling out for them, responding with weeping and disorganized behavior to unfamiliar caregivers. They estimated that in a typical night, they had to help her with toileting at least once after she called for them.

In anticipation of a much-needed 5-day vacation, they asked their general internist for guidance about how to help her manage better in their absence. One of her other daughters was willing to care for her while they were away. To induce sleep, the doctor recommended a complicated psychotropic regimen that included zolpidem 5 mg or amitriptyline 25 mg at bedtime. For agitation during the day, the doctor recommended either 2 mg of haloperidol or 1 mg of lorazepam up to three times a day.

The first night her usual caregivers were away, she had difficulty falling asleep and was given both zolpidem and amitriptyline. A few hours later, she woke up disoriented and fell out of bed. She did not seem to recognize her daughter, who responded to the thump as she hit the floor and to her yelling. The daughter gave her a dose of lorazepam, and when she seemed to become even more agitated, followed it up with haloperidol that eventually appeared to calm her. She napped for much of the next day, and the same series of events with the same medication regimen occurred three out of the four subsequent nights.

When her daughter and son-in-law returned from their vacation, they found the patient confused, with "waxing and waning" alertness, impressive stiffness in her limbs and trunk, and prominent tremors, particularly on her right side. She had been eating and drinking poorly since they had left, and they decided to take her to the emergency department of their local hospital. On examination, she was determined to be dehydrated and delirious with a possible urinary tract infection and was admitted to the hospital for observation and treatment.

◆ **Diagnosis: Axis I—Delirium, 293.0; Rule Out Dementia Not Otherwise Specified, 294.8**

This case illustrates the dangers of polypharmacy in the elderly for dementia-related problems. In particular, given the history of possible Parkinson's disease, it points up the inappropriate use of haloperidol in parkinsonian patients, who are very prone to extrapyramidal side effects from antipsychotic agents (particularly high-potency first-generation antipsychotic agents). In addition, it is probable that the patient experienced disinhibition from lorazepam and that her baseline tenuous cognition was affected by anticholinergic side effects of amitriptyline.

Patients with neurodegenerative conditions have compromised "cerebral reserve" and as such are prone to delirium when given anticholinergics and benzodiazepines. Complicating the picture, high-potency antipsychotics, by virtue of their robust blockade of dopamine receptors, may acutely exacerbate parkinsonian symptoms.

In a broader context, this dementia patient had been behaviorally stable in the family home with familiar caretakers and a predictable routine. Perhaps she had difficulty with sleep onset as part of a "catastrophic reaction" due to the disruption in her care model, which she may not have understood as only temporary. The onset of disruption of her behavior at night, a time of relative sensory deprivation, may have been potentiated by her chronic vision and hearing impairment. The insomnia led to the unfortunate cascade of psychopharmacological events that led to an episode of delirium.

When assessing acute altered mental status, particularly in elderly patients, prompt review of recently ingested medications, sleep disturbance, and changes in the social environment should be assessed in parallel. In addition, screening for urinary tract infection and other infectious diseases should be routinely accomplished. In Parkinson's disease (either established or suspected), the use of high-potency first-generation antipsychotics is fraught with danger. If sedation is clinically necessary, second-generation antipsychotic agents with low dopamine blockade activity (e.g., quetiapine) may be tried, because they are less likely to exacerbate parkinsonian symptoms.

Frontal Oligoastrocytoma With Abulia

A 58-year-old white man with a history of hypertension and degenerative joint disease had a single generalized seizure that led to the discovery of a left frontal oligoastrocytoma. This lesion was resected the previous year, followed by x-ray therapy and chemotherapy. He returned to the hospital and underwent a second surgical exploration because it appeared that his tumor had recurred. The surgery revealed this concern to have been a false alarm.

The patient said he was puzzled that psychiatry had been consulted. He was aware that his physiatrist had suggested he visit with a neuropsychologist to review recent neurocognitive testing in detail, but he had no explanation for our involvement. The patient's wife then chimed in to say that she was responsible for initiating the request because she was frustrated by the change in the patient's personality in recent months.

The patient said that he had been content since his initial surgery and was unaware of any particular concern. He acknowledged he displayed little initiative and was now content to watch television and play solitaire throughout much of the day, in contrast to the years prior to discovery of his tumor when he was much more apt to be found outside working on various projects. The patient related he did not enjoy news programs anymore, but he still watched old movies and played solitaire (a perseverative detail in the interview). His ability to concentrate and follow along during a news show was subjectively impaired, but he felt he had no difficulty following the plot in most movies. He denied self-denigrating thoughts or any thoughts of being less worthwhile, even though his life has become much more sedentary and less goal oriented. He firmly denied dysphoria or depression. He denied suicidal ideation. He reiterated that he felt content and comfortable with his current existence in a remote, rural part of his state.

The patient presented as a quiet individual with a slight lisp in his slow, deliberate speech. His thought processes were generally linear, and his mood was euthymic. He demonstrated a persistent and somewhat superficial "all is well" demeanor. He denied suicidal ideation. His insight was concrete, but his judgment was appropriate for the conduct of this interview.

The patient was born and raised in Oklahoma, and after graduation from high school he began to work as a pipe fitter. He married early in adulthood but never had children. After working in a variety of Midwestern states, he settled in a large urban area, working in maintenance at a manufacturing plant. He had retired not long before the discovery of his tumor. The patient and his wife moved to a distant resort area where they lived year-round in a trailer. They had limited social interaction because the community was populated only on weekends and then by people with other social networks.

The patient's wife commented on his tendency to withdraw socially. Even on those occasions when they went out, he was much more inclined to sit quietly and eat or appear to simply observe conversation without participating. She noted that he seemed perpetually complacent, and this frustrated her because she believed it was indicative of depression. She contrasted his behavior with the challenges she had faced after her own right-sided brain injury following a motor vehicle accident. She emphatically declared she had "exactly the same injury" and added that she overcame her deficits by sheer determination and practiced persistence. She also eventually acknowledged that she was a "city girl" and that she had become thoroughly exasperated by life in the isolated resort area where they had retired. She said she would love to move back to the city but then seemed to catch herself and hastily added that this would provide more social interaction and stimulation for her husband. At the conclusion of the consultation, when the psychiatrist's hand was reaching for the door, she asked directly, "Do you agree that daily stimulation will be important for Earl? I think it is medically essential for his rehabilitation that we move back to the city."

◆ Diagnosis: Axis I—Cognitive Disorder Not Otherwise Specified, 294.9

The consultation for this patient reminds us that multiple parties and agendas may prompt or shape the request. The psychiatrist later learned that the physiatrist had intended only to ask for a neuropsychology consultation to interpret the cognitive testing results for the patient. However, the patient's wife told the resident that her husband was "severely depressed, and I expect him to see a psychiatrist." She implied the attending had promised to arrange this detail.

Although the patient was not clinically depressed, he displayed features of abulia consistent with the location of his tumor and the anatomic consequences of its resection. This enabled the psychiatrist to educate the patient's wife about this condition, possible treatment strategies, and likely prognosis. Bupropion and other dopaminergic agonists may stimulate some improvement in initiative and activity among these patients, but the degree of response is often limited. A frequent complicating factor, as with this patient, is that these individuals may have a concomitant seizure disorder arising from whatever pathology precipitated the abulia.

The neurocognitive testing results provided further opportunity to help the spouse understand some of the reasons for the behaviors that frustrated her (e.g., his relative disinterest in rapid-flowing conversation when they were out in public) and also to capitalize on the fact that he would likely do much better with written and visual instructions and cues than with verbal learning. Unfortunately, the patient's wife was not receptive to this information and appeared to dismiss it, citing her own experience as more authoritative. Observing this unexpected reaction, the psychiatrist suspected that the wife's primary purpose in securing the consultation had little to do with concern about the patient's mood but may have had a great deal to do with her own deteriorating mood in the secluded setting of their retirement retreat.

Neurofibromatosis With Delirium, Depressed Mood, and Death

A 53-year-old man with neurofibromatosis, secondary hydrocephalus with a history of multiple shunts and subsequent revisions, seizure disorder, and intraspinal schwannomas was admitted to the hospital after a recurrent generalized seizure.

The previous year had been difficult. A year earlier, persistent severe headaches had led to the discovery that one of his three shunts was embedded in a pseudopancreatic cyst. His headaches improved but did not resolve after this was surgically corrected. Nine months later, he developed nausea with recurrent emesis and a new severe, constant headache. He was admitted to the neurosurgery service for externalization of his ventricular peritoneal shunts. However, after externalization of one shunt, he became delirious. A head computed tomography (CT) scan showed extensive edema surrounding the occipital and temporal horns. Externalization of a second shunt uncovered purulent drainage. Laboratory examination of his cerebrospinal fluid was remarkable for 7,070 white blood cells per mm³, glucose of 50 mg/dL, protein of 485 mg/dL, and multiple gram-negative rods and a few gram-positive bacilli. He had a generalized tonic-clonic seizure, and a repeat head CT revealed a new enhancing lobule in the left parieto-occipital lobe proximate to a catheter and suspicious for an abscess. Apart from infrequent lip-smacking, he had no further seizure activity after initiation of intravenous antibiotics and achieving a therapeutic level of phenytoin. A culture from the catheter tip grew *Klebsiella*. The patient improved as antibiotics were continued and, after an appropriate interval, a fourth ventricular pleural shunt and a right occipital pleural shunt were placed. He did well, with improved mental status, and tentative plans were made for transfer to a long-term physical rehabilitation unit.

Before this could be arranged and without a clear precipitant, the patient became less interactive and progressively uninterested in his meals and family visits. He retreated into a mute and seemingly solitary state despite the absence of any acute changes in laboratory parameters or on an electroencephalogram. He had had two prior bouts of depression, the most recent having been about 21 months earlier after being placed on medical disability. Duloxetine was associated with gradual improvement, and it had been discontinued after 12 months.

Psychiatry was consulted to assess for depression. Ironically, he was markedly more interactive during the psychiatry interview. He offered appropriate eye contact, and although there was a mild latency of response in his speech, the volume was appropriate and his rate was only slightly decreased. There was very little prosodic variation. His answers were succinct and indicated linear thought processes. There was no overt evidence of a formal thought disorder. He denied feeling depressed in mood and appeared generally euthymic to the examiner. His affect was bland apart from a tendency to smile reflexively whenever the interviewer smiled, regardless of the associated topic or expected affect. There were no other examples of echopraxia or evidence of stimulus-bound behavior. He was cognitively impaired, correctly naming the hospital he was in but doing so in a wooden voice and going on to say that his home was only a few minutes' drive away, rather than the actual 2-plus hours. The psychiatric team did not recommend initiation of an antidepressant but suggested repeat antiepileptic serum levels, which proved unremarkable.

The patient rallied inexplicably over the following day, even to the point of regaining his orientation and conversing appropriately with his family. He was able to walk for a short distance with the

assistance of his sons but then became increasingly quiet that afternoon and was observed to have frequent "staring spells." An electroencephalogram revealed sharp waves consistent with epileptic
activity. Plans were made to transfer him to the epilepsy monitoring
unit for continuous electroencephalographic recording while adjustments were made to his antiepileptic regimen. However, by the
following morning, he had again become mute, lethargic, and no
longer tolerated any oral intake due to persistent nausea and occasional emesis. Another head CT revealed marked dilatation of his
fourth ventricle, consistent with failure of the fourth ventricular
shunt.

A multidisciplinary team met with the patient's wife (a dermatologist) and his two siblings. The patient's family described multiple
previous discussions with the patient, particularly over the past
3 months, in which he had asked his wife to exercise her best judgment in choosing a time to refrain from further surgical interventions or other life-sustaining measures such as intravenous hydration or a feeding tube. The patient's wife and siblings concluded that
the patient would not want any further effort beyond comfort measures. His nausea and pain were aggressively addressed, and he was
discharged to a hospice near his home. He succumbed within the
week.

♦ **Diagnosis: Axis I—Delirium, 293.0; Major Depressive
Disorder, Recurrent, Severe Without Psychotic Features,
296.33**

This case illustrated elements of two common consultation dilemmas. The first is the importance of discerning the presence of hypoactive delirium in patients who may generate a consultation request
for nondescript "depression." This may be especially difficult in
cases in which the patient has had episodes of depression in the past.
The second is how to assess for depression in the context of a medical
illness that could reasonably account for multiple neurovegetative
signs and symptoms. Patients with central nervous system (CNS) lesions such as this case may be at risk for cognitive and mood symptoms. It may be difficult to diagnose a "pure" mood disorder in the
context of CNS cancer, even in a patient with a history of depression
episodes premorbidly. In addition, patients with a frontal lobe tumor
may have clinical findings consistent with apathy and/or catatonia-
spectrum symptoms as well.

Pathological Gambling, Bipolar Disorder, and Pramipexole

The patient was a 48-year-old married man with early-onset idiopathic Parkinson's disease. He was started on carbidopa/levodopa, with a dopamine agonist—pramipexole—added to help modulate his somewhat robotic motor movements. Over several months the dosage was advanced to 1.5 mg three times a day, and he tolerated the pramipexole without apparent side effects.

He had no known psychiatric history, although ever since a Native American casino opened up not far from his home, he had enjoyed going there several times a year to play blackjack and to take advantage of the inexpensive dinner buffet. Suddenly, after beginning pramipexole, seemingly in a matter of weeks, his appetite for gambling became insatiable. He drove to the casino on an almost daily basis and had over a period of several months wagered away his entire savings of $22,000. In addition, whereas before he and his wife had enjoyed making love once a week or so, he had become sexually aggressive to the point of demanding intercourse from his wife several times a day and becoming verbally threatening if she did not submit to his demands. Formerly indifferent to yard work, he had also become preoccupied with maintaining the cleanliness of his driveway and patio and spent at least 3 hours a day mopping and sweeping them.

Increasingly distraught by her husband's new series of behaviors, the patient's wife told their family doctor about the gambling and the incessant sexual demands. The family physician then made a psychiatric referral. The psychiatrist diagnosed pathological gambling and possible bipolar disorder, recommended that the patient begin attending Gamblers Anonymous meetings, and prescribed an atypical neuroleptic, olanzapine, to see if it would reduce the intensity of the gambling and sexual urges. Neither the patient nor his wife complained about his new-found devotion to patio care.

At his annual neurology follow-up, the neurologist observed that the patient had gained 15 pounds and noted that he was taking a "new medication," olanzapine, for what the patient told him was "bipolar disorder" that had suddenly "come on" since his last visit to the neurologist. Although he was by then less interested in gambling, he continued to push his wife for daily sexual activity, sulking if she did not give in. The neurologist confirmed the interval history with the patient's wife, who mentioned in passing his unusual devotion to the patio. Having read a recent case series on compulsive behaviors induced by dopamine agonists, the neurologist decided to taper the pramipexole over the next several months. On follow-up 6 months later, the patient could now "take or leave" visiting a casino, agreed that weekly intercourse is "plenty for a guy of my age," and seemed not to care that dirt and leaves had accumulated on the patio.

◆ **Diagnosis: Axis I—Adverse Effects of Medication Not Otherwise Specified, 995.2**

When evaluating and managing patients with neurological illness who also evidence active psychiatric symptoms, the challenge to the psychosomatic medicine psychiatrist is often one of accurate attribution. Neurological illnesses, such as Parkinson's disease in this man's case, are well known to be independently associated with psychiatric symptoms. This connection between neurological illness and psychiatric illness is quite clear if the clinician understands "neurological" illness as being evidence of a degenerative process of the CNS. There is little reason to believe that the "psychiatric" part of the brain should be somehow protected from the degenerative process affecting the "neurological" parts. In clinical practice, therefore, one commonly sees the psychiatric symptoms of anxiety, depression, and dementia in patients with Parkinson's disease as a "psychiatric" complication of a "neurological" illness. Better, perhaps, one can consider this whole spectrum of illness as "neuropsychiatric" disorders.

In addition, there is the independent comorbidity of psychiatric and neurological illness. Whether the new onset of a psychiatric syndrome in a neurological patient may be the understandable behavioral result of the clearly profound stress of managing a progressive and relentless illness, or whether the patient may have had psychiatric illness long before the onset of the neurological illness, in such a case one can postulate the two syndromes as developing along more independent tracks.

Finally, as in this case, the possibility is always lurking that the medications to treat neurological illness may themselves induce psychiatric syndromes. It is well known that dopaminergic Parkinson's disease medications may induce delusions and hallucinations as a result of modulation of the dopamine system. In this gentleman's case, the sequence of events led to the expression of symptoms suggesting a combination of pathological gambling and bipolar disorder. Once the connection between these symptoms and their temporal relationship to the use of pramipexole was established, the behavioral symptoms improved promptly with its discontinuation. Notably, the *Physician's Desk Reference* (2007) states that "cases of pathological gambling, hypersexuality, and compulsive eating (including binge eating) have been reported in patients treated with dopamine agonist therapy, including pramipexole therapy. As described in the literature, such behaviors are generally reversible upon dose reduction or treatment discontinuation" (p. 860).

Paraplegia and "Hyper-Sublimation"

The psychosomatic medicine psychiatrist often sees patients facing numerous and profound challenges to permanent and disabling conditions. Often the challenge is to treat a depressed and newly motor-impaired patient who must quickly adapt to the challenges of a rigorous physical rehabilitation program so as to optimize function, even though the new functional endpoint is a far lower level of function than the patient has been accustomed to. Added to these challenges is the fact that many trauma victims are young and invested in their physical selves as narcissistic objects; the acute sense of loss can be profound and enduring.

> The patient was a 27-year-old white man for whom a consultation was requested for "depression." Ten years earlier, he had been a high school track athlete, quite skilled at middle distances in track and field. He was poised to pursue a track and field scholarship in college when he was involved in a motor vehicle accident while in high school. As a result, he was permanently paraplegic and wheelchair bound. He was also required to self-catheterize and was prone to urinary tract infections. He had become depressed about the course of his illness and because the illness kept him from his job. He then proceeded to tell us an inspiring story of adaptation to his paraplegia, a story of "hyper-compensation."
>
> Following his accident and initial rehabilitation, he acutely mourned his loss of motor function. After all, even more than normative for a young man, this was a man whose identity was centered on physical prowess. After his initial rehabilitation, he became very involved in wheelchair athletics. His specialty was wheelchair marathon. Sometime later, he was (briefly) a record holder in the wheelchair marathon. Academically, he pursued a doctoral degree in exercise physiology. Once he was finished with graduate school, he obtained a position at a local university, where a major role was

being the academic and personal advisor to the disabled students on campus.

As he patiently explained, his depression was not simply due to the loss of his motor function. When he was home and at his university job and participating in wheelchair-based sports, he did not feel depressed at all. It was when his recurrent urinary tract infections and their complications required hospitalization, thus separating him from his life role, that he developed mood symptoms. This man's response to his tragic loss must have served as a powerful example to his student advisees.

◆ **Diagnosis: Axis I—Depressive Disorder Not Otherwise Specified, 311; Axis II—Narcissistic Traits**

Narcissistic personality, whether the full disorder or only traits, is commonly encountered in work with trauma patients. This may be due to a number of factors. In terms of risk for trauma in the first place, grandiose, self-confident, and reckless patients are more likely to take physical risks with various kinds of physical activity. In addition, the well-appreciated association between narcissistic personality and substance abuse can potentiate the risk for trauma by exposure to driving while intoxicated and other substance-related high-risk activity. Once injured and hospitalized, it is likely that narcissistic patients will frequently come into conflict with their caregivers and thus manifest conflict within the medical center care model. This therapeutic impasse and failure of the physician–patient relationship may lead to the need (often with urgency) for psychosomatic medicine consultation. Finally, grandiose, vain, and self-referential patients may be particularly distressed at having to deal with physical impairment. It is hard, to say the least, to fully integrate a narcissistic worldview (wherein the self is powerful, the object of envy, and omnipotent) with the depressing realities of one's newly acquired, often disfiguring, and functionally impairing injuries. No wonder, then, that the psychosomatic medicine consultant will frequently be called on to deal with narcissistic trauma victims who are indeed quite depressed, and maybe even suicidal, when confronting acute physical impairment and the need for active rehabilitation.

Once initial adjustment to loss has been managed, however, narcissistic personality may ironically confer some advantages on the rehabilitation task. Although there is a need for bargaining and compromise, the narcissistic patient (as in this case) may be able to invest in rehabilitation as a narcissistic object. In this way, rehabilitation itself becomes the object of identity and even vanity. The narcissistic patient may be motivated to mobilize physical resources to devote to rehabilitation, both to "show" the treating staff how they may have "underestimated" him with a limited prognosis and/or, more likely, to mobilize internal grandiosity to prove to the self that "I still can be grandiose, just in a different way." We propose the term "narcissistic hyper-sublimation" for this phenomenon. Surely this man demonstrated this applied concept.

Conversion Disorder (Plus)

The patient was a 24-year-old white man from a Southern rural background. He was an airman in the U.S. Air Force. During an outdoor drill at his base on a hot summer day, he collapsed. Taken to a regional military hospital, he was found to have weakness in his left lower extremity and underwent magnetic resonance imaging (MRI) that showed a small lesion of indeterminate focus in the pons. Upon hearing the news that his MRI scan was positive, he immediately developed paralysis from the neck down, with a demarcation line circumferentially around his neck. He was promptly transferred to a tertiary care medical center for a neurological workup that included psychosomatic medicine psychiatric consultation.

The psychiatrist's examination found a young, healthy-appearing man lying in bed with no spontaneous movements of his limbs or trunk. He had an animated expression on his face and described, with apparent indifference bordering on pleasure, the circumstances under which he found himself to be hospitalized. He stated that he came from a family in which the tradition of military service was strong across multiple generations. Although he would have preferred to train as a chef after graduating from high school, he had immediately enlisted in the Air Force "to maintain the family honor" and found himself instead working as a hospital orderly, a role that he detested. He wondered aloud—without any particular emotional overlay—whether his injury and functional impairment would result in his discharge from the Air Force on medical grounds.

Having been told by the neurology service that the distribution of the paralysis had no known anatomical correlation, particularly with the MRI finding, the psychiatrist concluded that a conversion disorder diagnosis was appropriate and recommended a rehabilita-

tive program that included intensive physical therapy and a psychotherapeutic approach that emphasized the temporary nature of the
disability and celebrated any signs of remission of the paralysis. The
patient was also encouraged to explore the conflict he had identified
between his family's expectations and his personal aspirations.

Over the next several weeks, physical therapy and psychotherapy
proceeded well, and the paralysis rapidly retreated until only mild
left-leg weakness remained. However, the patient's progress pla-
teaued until he acutely developed a new onset of unilateral optic
neuritis. On repeat MRI, additional cerebral lesions were noted, and
he was given the final diagnosis of multiple sclerosis.

◆ Diagnosis: Axis I—Conversion Disorder, 300.11

The phenomenon of conversion disorder, wherein a psychological conflict is "converted" into a physical symptom (which is often
symbolically representative of the underlying conflict) has been recognized for well over a century. Because the presentation of the patient is often focused on the apparent physical deficit, these cases will
often present primarily in a general or specialty (such as neurology,
in this case) medical context rather than a primary psychiatric one.
As such, it is likely that psychosomatic medicine psychiatrists are
more likely to see these cases than psychiatrists practicing in other
clinical models.

In this man's case, the initial diagnosis of conversion disorder was
completely consistent with the majority of the clinical facts at hand.
His likely intrapsychic conflict can be understood as related to his career development, a task that, for many young adults, occurs at the
time of establishing one's own residence and adult identity in more
general terms. This man had personal aspirations of becoming a
chef, yet there was a palpable family expectation of military service.
This alone may be an adequate substrate for intrapsychic conflict for
some, but his military career field as a hospital orderly further exacerbated the sense of conflict between his own goals and the voca-
tional situation in which he found himself.

His clinical presentation of physical collapse following exertion in
a training exercise is consistent with the formulation of conversion
disorder as well. Were he to be physically unable to adapt to military
service, this could have provided for an "allowable" way out of his
enlistment, perhaps thus allowing him to pursue career pathways

that were more resonant to him. The initially "incidental" MRI finding generating a catastrophic motor loss only potentiates this hypothesis.

The usual behavioral management of conversion disorder emphasized the hopeful stance, with focus on gradual "giving up" of the physical symptom over time and concurrent psychotherapeutic attention to conflict identification and solution. Such an approach was initiated in this man's case as well, with the initial gradual improvement one would usually expect in a conversion disorder case.

Only after the plateauing of improvement (as opposed to complete symptoms remission) did the case formulation lead one to explicitly expect more than "pure conversion" disorder. Unfortunately, the classic symptom of unilateral optic neuritis led to further evaluation with repeated neuroimaging, now showing multiple CNS lesions. A diagnosis of multiple sclerosis, although arrived at well after initial presentation, is at this point quite obvious.

This case illustrates a certain ambiguity. Had the patient experienced complete symptom relief with the initial intervention, and had he not later developed optic neuritis, this would have been in every way rather a classic conflict-driven case of pseudoneurological conversion disorder. From the retrospective side, with multiple CNS lesions evolving over time on neuroimaging and the ominous unilateral optic neuritis, the diagnosis of multiple sclerosis is equally clear.

When treating conversion disorder, one should always keep in mind the possibility of an eventual diagnosis of neurological illness or other systemic illness to enter the picture. Even if there is eventually a picture of a neurological illness as in this case, this does not mean per se that the initial conversion disorder was "wrong" as long as it is independently supportable; the fact is that cases are complex, and patients may migrate over time along a conceptual "psychiatric and neurological" continuum.

Decisional Capacity and Cultural Issues in a Neurosurgery Patient

A 68-year-old Cambodian man with a history of coronary artery disease, hypertension, hyperlipidemia, remote history tuberculosis, and latent syphilis presented to the hospital due to several months of progressive weakness in his right upper extremity. He chose to come to the hospital when he noticed that he was finding it increasingly difficult to hold his neck upright and that swallowing no longer seemed automatic and effortless.

A female friend accompanying the patient said that in the past 2 weeks his behavior had changed, characterized by episodes of inappropriate laughter and apparent disorientation. Following an extensive workup including head CT, carotid ultrasound, electroencephalography, electromyelography, cervical MRI, dobutamine stress echocardiography, bilateral lower extremity ultrasound, and a variety of serologic tests, the patient was diagnosed with cervical myelopathy. He was advised that there would be reasonable hope of achieving substantial relief from his symptoms with surgical intervention, but he declined to consent to this procedure. Psychosomatic medicine psychiatry was asked to assess whether he had the capacity to make an informed decision on this issue.

With the assistance of a Cambodian interpreter, the patient was able to describe his medical condition in general terms, including an appreciation for his coronary artery disease and his understanding that a "pinched nerve" was responsible for his right upper extremity symptoms. He said he was not aware of any known therapeutic alternatives to the proposed surgery. He declined to answer when asked about the risks and benefits of the proposed surgery, preferring to repeat several times that he did not believe it would be helpful. He explained that he believed his destiny mandated that he carry on in his present condition. He volunteered that he understood that he would eventually die but added that he would receive no benefit from the surgery and then would also face death, so he could see no differential merit in accepting the recommended surgery.

He clarified his conviction regarding the lack of benefit from the proposed surgery by saying that "they" had instructed him that surgery would not be helpful and that he must not consent. After further pursuit, he described "they" as a constellation of "spirits" who cared for him and whom he was able to see in the room as the interview proceeded. He acknowledged that these spirits were also speaking to him in the midst of the conversation with the psychiatrist, and they were increasingly advising him to be wary and disclose little of either what they said to him or what he was thinking.

Having shared this, the patient became progressively less interactive and ultimately declined to answer any further questions. Prior to completely withdrawing and embracing a mute state, the patient shared that he would receive punishment from the spirits if he consented to the proposed surgery, although he was not willing to detail what these adverse consequences might be. He frowned and rejected the suggestion that it was possible that the spirits and his physicians might collaborate for his benefit. He did not respond when asked why it was that, although he perceived these spirits were intent upon caring for him, they had apparently chosen to require him to suffer with the disabilities that he was currently experiencing and were not allowing him to pursue relief of these symptoms. Similarly, he declined to comment when the examiner asked him to help the examiner understand why it was that his female friend stated that these changes in thought patterns have only occurred over the past month. The examiner also gingerly inquired whether it was possible that these "spirits" reflected another illness; the patient did not respond.

The patient was lying on his hospital bed on his right side with a small towel drawn over his eyes because he complained that he found light irritating. He spoke freely with the interpreter at the outset of the interview and appeared to generally offer linear thought processes. As the interview proceeded, he became progressively less responsive to the point where he ultimately simply lay quietly without offering any verbal or nonverbal response. His mood appeared sober and subdued but not melancholic. When he first began to laugh in a silent and curious manner, it was difficult to discern whether he was crying or laughing because his facial musculature, although active, was ambiguous. However, over time, it became more apparent that this was laughing and not crying. He denied suicidal ideation and said the spirits had never asked him to do anything explicitly self-harmful. He refused to answer questions about orientation or other domains of cognitive function, but his description of his medical history and condition was accurate.

♦ **Diagnosis: Axis I—Rule Out Acculturation Problem, V62.4; Rule Out Psychotic Disorder Not Otherwise Specified, 298.9**

The Cambodian interpreter advised the psychiatrist that there is a small subset of Cambodian Buddhists who subscribe to the existence of a spirit world ruled by the "Master" and who commonly relate that they are able to see and hear these spirits. The Cambodian interpreter further noted that there is an especially devout but even more minuscule number of this subset who consistently refuse all medical care of any kind throughout life, because they believe it is the sole responsibility of these spirits to exercise healing. The interpreter added that it is commonplace for these individuals to speak quite openly about their ability to see and hear these spirits, although she found the character of the patient's periodic laughter peculiar and beyond any cultural explanation familiar to her.

The psychiatrist advised the neurosurgical team that the patient was either unable or unwilling to consistently demonstrate the capacity for independent decision making in his own best interest. Despite successfully relating a passably factual understanding of his medical condition and remaining steady in his refusal to accept the proposed surgery, the patient had also repeatedly declined to cooperate with cognitive screening exercises designed to assess his mental ability.

Although the rejection of surgery appeared, at first glance, to be rooted in a psychotic or parapsychotic experience (particularly in light of the friend's account that the patient's behavior had changed in the previous month), it was difficult to make this assertion with unambivalent confidence. The interpreter had opened a window on a religious and cultural context that provided a rationale for the patient's choice. In the absence of compelling collateral evidence that the patient's perspective was distorted by depression or a primary psychotic illness, the psychiatrist concluded this was an unusual situation in which, despite the absence of a convincing demonstration of cognitive capacity, there were sufficient and complex extenuating circumstances that warranted caution before pursuing legal approval for the proposed treatment contrary to the patient's expressed wishes. In some institutions, a clinical dilemma with competing priorities prompts further consultation from a designated ethics consultation service that allows for additional multidisciplinary reflection before settling on a course of action.

Asperger's Disorder Presenting in Late Life: A Diagnostic Dilemma

Case 1

A 70-year-old white man, found walking unsteadily on the grounds of a local high school, was brought by police to the emergency department of a university medical center. He was diagnosed with diabetic ketoacidosis and hypertensive encephalopathy and admitted to a general medical service. His acute disorientation quickly improved with treatment of his systemic medical problems, but the patient continued to appear "odd" to the primary medical team, and it was believed that he might have dementia. The psychosomatic medicine service was asked to see this patient to evaluate his decisional capacity to make placement decisions. The primary team had recommended that the patient move into a board and care supervised placement, where he would be provided with meals and medication, whereas the patient had a rather vague plan of "getting back my RV."

Prior to admission, the patient had spent the previous 20 years of his life traveling between northern and southern parts of the state in his recreational vehicle (RV). During this time, he had been able to care for his diabetes mellitus and acquire his own food. He received a monthly disability income that was adequate to obtain his basic needs. In the weeks prior to his hospital admission, the patient had run into difficulties trying to acquire insulin without a prescription (his physician had retired, and he had not obtained follow-up care), and he had been pulled over by the police on several occasions for erratic driving. As a result of police interventions, his RV was impounded and his driver's license suspended. He had no relatives or friends with whom he regularly communicated, although the social services department, upon inquiry, did uncover that the patient had previously been cared for by his sister until her death 20 years earlier. He had no prior formal psychiatric history, but distant relatives did report lifetime problems with school and work performance.

The patient's mental status examination was notable for his cooperation despite considerable social awkwardness. He rarely made eye contact and would use odd gestures that would remain fixed for unusually long intervals. His thought process was tangential and perseverative on the theme of getting his RV back. He had no psychotic or mood symptoms. He was neither suicidal nor homicidal. He scored 28 on the Mini-Mental State Examination (MMSE; Folstein et al. 1975) and was able to generate 15 words in 60 seconds on categories testing. His clock drawing test was normal.

In evaluating the patient's ability to make placement decisions, the psychosomatic medicine team applied the Applebaum and Grisso (1988) method of capacity determinations and found that although the patient appeared to understand his medical diagnoses, he did not fully appreciate the risks of going untreated. This patient appeared unable to grasp that his RV was impounded or that he was no longer in possession of a driver's license, and as a result he was essentially functionally homeless. He was unable to adjust to new circumstances and formulate a reasonable placement care plan for himself. A surrogate decision maker agreed to send the patient to a board and care placement where he would receive assistance with medications, transportation to appointments, and all his meals.

This case brought up strong feelings in house staff and attending physicians on the internal medicine service, who had strongly positive countertransferential feelings for the patient and wanted him to continue "roaming the state" in the manner he seemed to enjoy. After discharge, a social services follow-up did confirm that the patient had adapted well to the board and care placement and was able to get appropriate medical follow-up appointments with support from board and care staff.

♦ **Diagnosis: Axis I—Rule Out Asperger's Disorder, 299.80; Rule Out Cognitive Disorder Not Otherwise Specified, 294.9; Axis II—Schizoid Traits**

Case 2

A 61-year-old white man presented to the emergency department at a university medical center with crushing substernal chest pain. After initial evaluation, he was found to have an acute myocardial infarction and critical stenosis of several coronary arteries. A coronary artery bypass graft procedure was recommended by the cardiothoracic surgery team. The patient initially refused surgery, stating that he "needed to take care of some personal business." Social services and psychosomatic medicine consultations were requested in view of the patient's homelessness, lack of social supports, "odd affect," and tangential speech. The cardiothoracic team questioned the patient's decisional capacity to consent to surgery.

On initial psychiatric evaluation, the patient appeared hypervigilant and was guarded when asked personal information. He reported having lived out of his car with no fixed address for many years and earning money doing odd jobs. His family lived across the country, and he had only infrequent contact with them. On mental status examination, the patient was noted to be wearing dark sunglasses while lying in an intensive care unit bed. He grimaced frequently. His mood was irritable, and his affect was somewhat blunted. He denied prior psychiatric symptoms or treatment, but he refused to give permission for collateral sources to be contacted. The patient scored 29 on the MMSE and generated 14 unique animals in 60 seconds in category testing. Regarding the recommended surgery, the patient reiterated his desire to "take care of some things" and return to the hospital for surgery at a later date. However, when he was confronted about the seriousness of his medical condition, the patient agreed to stay and have surgery. After this consultation, the team felt that he had the decisional capacity to accept the graft operation. The psychiatry psychosomatic medicine team recommended avoiding high-potency antipsychotics due to possible tardive dyskinesia (which was suggested by his symptom of grimacing) and the use of a low dose of olanzapine (2.5 mg) for any paranoia and agitation. His initial diagnosis was "rule out schizophrenia, paranoid type" and schizoid/paranoid personality traits.

Five days after surgery, the psychiatry service was now asked to evaluate the patient's decisional capacity to make placement decisions. On this interview, the patient was unable to formulate a reasonable plan to provide food, clothing, and shelter after hospitalization. His MMSE score was now 21, and he appeared to have impaired attention and disorganized thought. Delirium was suspected, and laboratory tests were ordered accordingly. Acute renal insufficiency and the postoperative use of opiate analgesics were implicated as contributing factors to his delirium. After the patient's renal function returned to normal and opiates were stopped, his MMSE increased to 28, and it appeared that his delirium was resolved. At this point, the patient was still unable to formulate a self-care plan, and he was discharged to an inpatient psychiatric facility on an involuntary psychiatric hold for grave disability.

◆ **Diagnosis: Axis I—Rule Out Asperger's Disorder, 299.80; Rule Out Schizophrenia, Undifferentiated Type, 295.90; Axis II—Schizoid Traits**

These two cases highlight some of the diagnostic and treatment challenges faced by physicians working with adult patients with evidence suggesting developmental disorders. Asperger's syndrome was first described by Hans Asperger (1944) and only reached greater recognition through the work of Lorna Wing (1981). Thus, older adults who may have this disorder likely went undiagnosed as children. The DSM-IV-TR diagnostic criteria can be seen in Table 14–1 (American Psychiatric Association 2000). Although the criteria exclude a diagnosis of Asperger's syndrome in those with problems in language and cognitive development, difficulties with pragmatic thought and oddities of speech have been described with Asperger's syndrome (Baron-Cohen et al. 1997). Baron-Cohen et al. (2005) have developed a new instrument for improving the diagnosis of Asperger's disorder in adults.

Both patients discussed in these examples were initially suspected of having psychiatric illnesses more often diagnosed in adult populations—dementia in the first patient and schizophrenia in the second. In the case of the first patient, he was initially thought to have a frontotemporal type of dementia, characterized by predominant

TABLE 14–1. DSM-IV-TR diagnostic criteria for Asperger's disorder.

A. Qualitative impairment in social interaction, as manifested by at least two of the following:

  (1) marked impairment in the use of multiple nonverbal behaviors such as eye-to-eye gaze, facial expression, body postures, and gestures to regulate social interaction

  (2) failure to develop peer relationships appropriate to developmental level

  (3) a lack of spontaneous seeking to share enjoyment, interests, or achievements with other people (e.g., by a lack of showing, bringing, or pointing out objects of interest to other people)

  (4) lack of social or emotional reciprocity

B. Restricted repetitive and stereotyped patterns of behavior, interests, and activities, as manifested by at least one of the following:

  (1) encompassing preoccupation with one or more stereotyped and restricted patterns of interest that is abnormal either in intensity or focus

  (2) apparently inflexible adherence to specific, nonfunctional routines or rituals

  (3) stereotyped and repetitive motor mannerisms (e.g., hand or finger flapping or twisting, or complex whole-body movements)

  (4) persistent preoccupation with parts of objects

C. The disturbance causes clinically significant impairment in social, occupational, or other important areas of functioning.

D. There is no clinically significant general delay in language (e.g., single words used by age 2 years, communicative phrases used by age 3 years).

E. There is no clinically significant delay in cognitive development or in the development of age-appropriate self-help skills, adaptive behavior (other than in social interaction), and curiosity about the environment in childhood.

F. Criteria are not met for another specific pervasive developmental disorder or schizophrenia.

Source. Reprinted from American Psychiatric Association: *Diagnostic and Statistical Manual of Mental Disorders*, 4th Edition, Text Revision. Washington, DC, American Psychiatric Association, 2000. Used with permission.

executive dysfunction. However, when a broader view of his lifelong isolation was considered, the change from baseline functioning required for a diagnosis of dementia could not be established. In the case of the second patient, eccentricities of dress and facial expression were initially taken to be signs of schizophrenia, but again, when placed in the context of his lifestyle, appeared to be part of a lifelong pattern consistent with Asperger's disorder.

Adults with Asperger's disorder may have poor connections to others (including family members) and rigid cognitive processes such that they are particularly unable to respond flexibly to changes in their personal circumstances. In both cases outlined, the patients had been functioning on the outskirts of society and taking care of their basic needs until several external factors conspired to make maintaining their previous lifestyles impossible. Both patients lacked social support, likely related to the impairments in social interaction related to Asperger's syndrome. Both patients demonstrated marked cognitive rigidity and an inability to adjust to "bumps in the road" caused by worsening/emerging medical illness. Thus, the psychosomatic medicine psychiatrist, encountering these patients in late life and in the context of systemic illness, was in a position to diagnose an illness usually thought of as a childhood-onset illness. These men grew up at a time when Asperger's syndrome was little recognized and might have benefited greatly from the social skills training and special academic training available to children diagnosed today.

Dementia With Preserved Motor Skills: The Long and Amnestic Journey Home

Dementia is, in most cases, an insidiously progressive disease of increasing cognitive and functional impairment. Often during the course of a dementia case, frank confrontation of the patient and his or her (often enabling) family members is necessary to curtail the patient's driving out of concerns for safety. There may be a great discrepancy between preservation of the more concrete and overlearned motor skills needed for driving (e.g., starting and operating the car, acquiring fuel and supplies, and recall of familiar routes) and the loss of ability to learn new material (anterograde amnesia) and progressively poor judgment due to dementia. The following case illustrates these points quite dramatically and points out the need for a clinical approach that addresses these issues in order to contain patients who should not be driving even when they retain some of the basic skills needed to do so.

The patient was a 75-year-old white man who was admitted to the medical center for evaluation of memory loss. The patient denied any difficulties with memory, but his family members (his wife and daughter) told a remarkable story that illustrated these concerns dramatically. The patient had a generally unremarkable medical and psychiatric history. He had retired several years earlier and lived a quiet life in the Midwest with his wife of 40 years. He continued to drive the family vehicle (because his wife had never liked driving and preferred that he continue to be the primary driver in the family) and had not been involved in traffic mishaps. His family (his daughter lived nearby and saw the patient and his spouse frequently) had noted the insidious onset of cognitive impairment. He had become prone to forgetting the names of even very familiar people, had a great deal of difficulty in learning the names of new people he met, and frequently would appear perplexed when asked simple questions. He would frequently pause in the middle of a household task, having forgotten what he was doing. His family members began to cover up for him; for example, they would provide the forgotten names of people for him, prompt him to finish household tasks, and supervise his activities on an essentially continuous basis. He did not receive medical evaluation for his cognitive impairment at this point. His wife continued to encourage him to drive, although either his wife or daughter would insist on accompanying him on all car trips to "be sure he doesn't get lost" and to offer navigational support. This arrangement, tenuous though it was, was continued for well over a year without any untoward events.

The patient, spouse, and daughter made frequent trips to Florida in the winter to escape the dreary Midwest for a more pleasant climate. For the many years that the family had been making this trip, the patient typically drove the entire distance. The same route was always followed, including a series of familiar fuel and rest stops along the way. Several months after the patient's cognitive deficits had become evident to his family, the three of them embarked yet again on their annual trip, with the impaired patient at the wheel and his family members accompanying him as they had been doing in the local area. They were cautious not to let him drive alone.

The trip from the Midwest to Florida was completed uneventfully. They established themselves at their vacation home as they had been doing for years. Despite his cognitive impairment, the patient, recognizing his familiar seasonal home, adapted to the routine in his new location. One morning, the patient's spouse and daughter went walking in the neighborhood, intending only a brief absence, leaving the patient, the car keys, and the vehicle at the vacation home. When they returned, they were horrified to find the patient and the vehicle gone. Initially hoping that he had, out of habit, driven to a local store, and perhaps minimizing the degree of his cognitive impairment, they did not contact law enforcement (had they done so, they would have had to admit their complicity in encouraging his driving in the first place).

When he did not return for several hours, they did not know what to do. They called some local friends in Florida, but none had seen him. Frantically, they called other family members back home in the Midwest seeking help. When he did not return home at all that day, one family member wondered if he had headed back to the Midwest. Still resisting calling law enforcement, one family member came up with an ingenious idea. The family called the credit card company and requested a report of charges on the patient's credit card use.

Supporting the family's suspicion, this search quickly revealed a series of new credit card charges for meals, fuel, and motel rooms in a northerly vector between Florida and the patient's home in the Midwest. He had simply headed home on his family's familiar route! Once his family realized what was happening, his wife and daughter hurriedly traveled home by airplane. Sure enough, he arrived in his driveway as expected. Finally motivated to seek evaluation of his cognitive impairment, his family immediately brought him to the medical center for evaluation. There were no incidents of his getting lost en route or of any motor vehicle accidents on this amnestic journey.

When clinically evaluated, the patient was unable to recall having been to Florida in the recent past (although he readily recalled that he "always went to Florida in the winter"). He admitted that yes, he still was driving, but that he did not recall having been on a long trip anytime recently. He was not psychotic and not agitated; in fact, he presented in a calm and pleasant, if somewhat vacant manner.

His formal cognitive examination revealed profound orientation, memory, and concentration impairment with relatively preserved language function and ability to communicate. Indeed, he appeared superficially to have normal social behavior, and had cognitive function not been formally tested, the profundity of his deficits could have been easily missed. His family, after relating the remarkable story of his solo return drive to the Midwest, was now able to take steps to provide 24-hour supervision and to keep him from driving permanently. CT scans of the head revealed global atrophy consistent with dementia. He was discharged to his family's care.

♦ **Diagnosis: Axis I—Dementia of the Alzheimer's Type, With Behavioral Disturbance, 294.11**

Dementia ultimately affects many areas of cognitive function, but by definition it must affect memory as a necessary element. This patient presented with a remarkable degree of amnesia, because he was unable to learn new material. However, he retained familiar motor skills as illustrated by his ability to drive and to use what could be called "overlearned survival skills" of using a credit card, operating a motor vehicle, and navigating a familiar route. The disparity between his amnesia and his ability to maintain these other skills (added to a clearly enabling stance by his family members) allowed him to continue to drive for far too long.

When confronted with his impairments, his family, chastened by their harrowing experience of fear for his safety on his long and solitary journey, now agreed to curtail his driving. Thankfully, a tragedy was averted. Clinicians will occasionally encounter cases of dementia patients who continue to drive when it is not cognitively safe to do so. This remarkable case illustrates, in a way, how far overlearned survival skills can be preserved long after other critical cognitive skills have been lost.

Movement Disorders and Dementia

There are many schemes available to classify dementing disorders, for example, cortical versus subcortical, acute onset versus insidious onset, reversible versus irreversible. Among the more useful clinically is a distinction based on the physical examination, because the psychiatric interview and formal mental status (including cognitive) testing may not be determinative (Marsh 2000; Rosenblatt and Leroi 2000). The distinction referred to is "dementia with a movement disorder" versus "dementia without a movement disorder." As in much of psychosomatic medicine (or much of the rest of medicine, for a sobering but necessary perspective), the apparent dichotomy of "with" and "without" is not an absolute one but may be perhaps better framed as "substantial" versus "no or unsubstantial" movement disorder. Because most of the "dementia with movement disorder" syndromes are progressive and degenerative neurological illnesses, the movement disorder may progress at a rate disconnected from progression of the cognitive impairment, so that later in the course of illness, movement disorder may be a more robust clinical covariate than when the patient first experienced cognitive symptoms.

With dementia cases, it is important to be aware of or to complete portions of the neurological clinical examination. Disorders of movement, such as tremor, choreathetoid movements, and impaired gait and station, are all to be considered. Dementia with a movement disorder is a large category, with many obscure dementia syndromes included. Some of the more classic or characteristic dementia syndromes associated with movement disorder include Parkinson's disease, Huntington's disease, multiple sclerosis, and prion disease (Marsh 2000; Rosenblatt and Leroi 2000).

Thus, the presence of a movement disorder at the outset of the course of clinical cognitive impairment leads the physician down the pathway of general neurodegenerative disease. The presentation of Lewy body dementia is more ambiguous; although it is not unusual to see associated movement disorder, patients do not have dramatic disorders of movement at diagnosis. Generally, the dementias due to primarily cortical pathology (e.g., Alzheimer's disease) and most cases of vascular dementia are not associated with disorders of movement, nor are some other dementia syndromes such as HIV dementia, dementia due to hypothyroidism, and dementia associated with traumatic brain injury (TBI).

Parkinson's Disease and Psychotic Depression

When treating patients with movement disorders for a wide range of psychiatric illnesses, it is important to remember that movement disorder symptoms may be exacerbated by the use of psychotropic agents. A tangible example is Parkinson's disease, which is associated with depression, psychosis, and dementia. However, treatment of psychosis in Parkinson's disease with antipsychotic medications can be associated with worsening of the underlying movement disorder; correspondingly, treatment of the movement disorder with dopaminergic medications can cause psychotic symptom exacerbation. Therefore, psychosomatic physicians treating Parkinson's disease patients on inpatient neurology services should routinely incorporate elements of the neurological examination into their clinical routine and remain vigilant for exacerbation of movement disorders as psychiatric symptoms improve. In addition, patients with movement disorders may be on medications that cause problematic drug–drug interactions, which can cause therapeutic dilemmas in managing cases.

The patient was an 80-year-old white man, a retired English teacher with a psychiatric history that was unremarkable until the recent past. In his mid-70s, he developed classic pill-rolling tremor and bradykinesia, leading to a diagnosis of Parkinson's disease. He had had a previous episode of depression, treated for several months with sertraline, early in the course of his Parkinson's disease. He had recently relocated to be closer to his middle-aged adult children. His Parkinson's disease motor symptoms had been under reasonable control with carbidopa/levodopa and selegiline (with residual tremor and bradykinesia that were not noticeably disruptive to his daily activities). He did not have a history of cognitive symptoms or impairment on examination.

Three weeks prior to being admitted to the hospital, he was driving near his home and was involved in a minor traffic accident. No one in either vehicle was injured, and damage to each vehicle was minimal. However, the patient shortly thereafter experienced an escalating series of delusions. Initially, he would ruminate on how the accident had really been much more serious than it appeared. Then, he became convinced that (due to his liability in causing the accident) he would be ruined financially and that his family would be made to suffer financially as well.

This delusion expanded progressively to the point that he believed distant family members across the country would suffer financial and legal ruin, again all because of him. During this time he also had a recurrence of his depression symptoms, with sadness, decreased energy, disinterest in familiar activities, and disturbance in his sleep and appetite. He attempted to run away from family members so that they "wouldn't be burdened by" having him in their lives.

Because his behavior had become unmanageable on an outpatient basis, he was admitted to the medical center for concurrent medical, neurological, and psychiatric evaluation. Upon examination he appeared mildly disheveled and bradykinetic, with small-amplitude pill-rolling tremor of both hands, equal bilaterally. His affect was dysphoric and blunted, and he became intermittently tearful when telling us how profoundly guilty he felt for having caused "ruin in so many family members' lives." He was not suicidal and not homicidal but remained delusional about his responsibility for the suffering of others. Despite his mood and psychotic symptoms, he was able to score 27 on the MMSE with some effort.

He was diagnosed with depression and psychosis, both due to Parkinson's disease. Herein were two dilemmas. His mood state was in need of treatment, but he continued to receive selegiline. Selegiline is a monoamine oxidase inhibitor, and thus is problematic to use concurrently with most antidepressant agents because a medically dangerous serotonin syndrome could result from their interaction. However, he had a history of treated depression and was currently profoundly depressed and psychotic.

The second dilemma was the usual one of how to manage psychosis in a patient with Parkinson's disease. Functionally, it is helpful to conceptualize Parkinson's disease (with its characteristic movement disorder) and psychosis on opposite ends of a "dopamine continuum." On the dopamine "depleted" end is Parkinson's disease, an illness of dopamine deficiency. On the dopamine "excessive activity" end are psychotic symptoms. Overlapping with this are the usual clinical interventions. Many Parkinson's disease symptoms are treated with carbidopa/levodopa to supplement the dopamine level in neural circuits. A common side effect of dopamine enhancement is emergence of psychosis. On the other end of the dopamine continuum, psychosis (modeled classically as a dopamine excess state) is treated with antipsychotic agents, which are dopamine D_2 blockers. Of course, a common side effect of typical antipsychotic agents is parkinsonism.

The first dilemma was addressed by discontinuing his selegiline. However, the washout period for selegiline—the time needed to eliminate the drug from the system sufficiently to allow safe use of serotonergic antidepressants—is 2 weeks. With no appropriate antidepressant option available during the washout period, attention focused on treating his psychosis. Because of his Parkinson's disease, it was important to choose, among the atypical antipsychotic agents, one with relatively less dopamine receptor blockade. The psychiatrist chose quetiapine, often considered to be the most tolerable atypical antipsychotic in Parkinson's disease. (Clozapine is similarly low in D_2 receptor blockade, but in an older patient is thought to be a significant delirium risk, and it was thus avoided.)

His quetiapine dosage was gently up-tapered during the period of selegiline washout. At a dose of 25 mg twice a day he was somewhat less delusional and less dysphoric; he was able to tolerate the quetiapine without noticeable increase in his movement disorder. Over the next 4 weeks, his quetiapine dosage was incrementally increased to 100 mg every morning and 175 mg every night, with some improvement in his delusional symptoms; gradual up-tapering of the dosage was tolerated without notable orthostatic hypotension or worsening of his dyskinesia.

After the 2-week washout of selegiline, he was begun on a low dosage of venlafaxine 37.5 mg extended release every morning; this was increased gradually to a dosage of 150 mg every morning. However, when the dosage of venlafaxine was increased beyond 150 mg daily, he began to have mild anticholinergic side effects, so the dosage was thereafter maintained at 150 mg daily. Mirtazapine was added to the venlafaxine, with gradually increasing dosages to 45 mg at bedtime. On the combination of quetiapine, venlafaxine, and mirtazapine, he showed periods of substantially less depressed mood and diminished psychotic symptoms while arrangements were made for electroconvulsive therapy (ECT). After his first six sessions of ECT, his mood was notably more improved, with no further delusional thinking, no suicidality, more spontaneous smiling, and an improved appetite. At that point, he was ready for discharge and outpatient care and was maintained on quetiapine, mirtazapine, and venlafaxine. He continued to receive his course of ECT as an outpatient.

◆ **Diagnosis: Axis I—Major Depressive Disorder, Recurrent, Severe With Psychotic Features, 296.34**

Parkinson's disease and its varied manifestations represent a particular challenge for psychosomatic medicine. Integration of evaluation of the motor aspects of the disease, both initially and progressively as the disease state changes, is important. The psychiatrist must be mindful that intervention for psychotic symptoms with antipsychotics may make movement disorder symptoms worse, whereas increased use of agents with dopaminergic activity to reverse movement disorder symptoms may be associated with psychosis as a complication. The physician must choose psychotropic agents thoughtfully to treat psychiatric symptoms while minimizing adverse motor symptoms. As illustrated in this case, awareness of drug–drug interactions must also guide treatment. ECT must be considered as a therapeutic option, both to accelerate improvement and to minimize exposure to medications.

Movement Disorder and Fronto-Subcortical Dementia: The Fragile X–Associated Tremor/Ataxia Syndrome

Fragile X syndrome is a leading cause of genetically determined, inherited mental retardation syndromes. In recent years, a new syndrome has been described in the premutation carriers for this syndrome. These patients do not have the full spectrum syndrome of fragile X but have been found to present in midlife and later with a combination of neurological symptoms (resting and intention tremor, ataxia and postural instability, and peripheral neuropathy) and psychiatric symptoms (anxiety, depression, and, most importantly, dementia). This condition is referred to as the fragile X–associated tremor/ataxia syndrome (FXTAS) (Hagerman and Hagerman 2004; Jacquemont et al. 2003). It is likely that some of these cases are misdiagnosed as Parkinson's disease with dementia, because the clinical appearances are similar. In addition to the very challenging combination of neurological and psychiatric symptoms these patients must deal with, there is often progression in impairments and significant functional impairment. In addition, once the pedigree analysis is completed, these patients may be consciously aware of (and even feel guilty about) being the "responsible party" for introducing the fragile X gene into their family and thus being indirectly "responsible" for the fragile X syndrome in their progeny.

A 55-year-old married white male electrician noted the insidious onset of tremor in his upper extremities. This progressed over a period of 4 years to the point that he had to retire from his job, a career at which he had been quite highly skilled and which had been a significant source of meaning for him. Over the next several years, the tremor intensified, and this previously independent man became dependent on others for assistance with most activities of daily living. He also developed ataxia and postural instability; empirical treatment with amantadine had briefly improved his postural status. He had two grandchildren with fragile X syndrome and a brother with fragile X syndrome and mental retardation.

When he received his first psychiatric evaluation 10 years after the onset of the neurological symptoms, his examination was notable for slowness of thought and laborious completion of simple motor tasks. He had excessive sleep, daytime naps, poor concentration, and notably slow psychomotor movements. His mood was irritably depressed, and his cognitive function was notable for poor recall of recent events and difficulty in recalling the names of close family members. His thought processes revealed perseveration with long latency of verbal responses. Affect was blunted and nontearful. His MMSE score was 24. An MRI revealed dilated cerebral ventricles and cortical atrophy. Genetic testing confirmed his fragile X premutation status. Formal neuropsychological testing revealed verbal IQ of 93, performance IQ of 73, and a full scale IQ of 83. Executive cognitive function was severely impaired, as were verbal fluency and processing speed.

He was diagnosed with FXTAS dementia and treated with donepezil, with the dosage titrated to 10 mg daily, and venlafaxine extended release 37.5 mg daily. With treatment, he had some initial improvement in short-term memory performance, improved sleep and energy, and better function in his activities of daily living. With this treatment, his psychiatric status showed stable improvement for more than 1 year. However, his tremors and ataxia progressed notably, and he became wheelchair bound and eventually bedridden. He died approximately 2.5 years after his initial psychiatric consultation, or 13 years after his onset of tremors.

◆ **Diagnosis: Axis I—Dementia Due to the Fragile X Tremor/Ataxia Syndrome, 294.11**

This syndrome, newly discovered, is associated with the premutation carrier state of the fragile X gene. Its discovery and initial descriptions were based on clinician observations of the family members of children with fragile X syndrome. Typically, it was noted that the grandfathers of fragile X children were developing first tremors, then later ataxia, and finally, in many cases, dementia. Only after these pedigrees were analyzed and genetic testing done on family members did it become clear that these grandfathers had the premutation carrier state that led, over subsequent generations, to the full syndrome in grandchildren.

Clinically, the physician may wish to consider a diagnosis of FXTAS dementia in cases of dementia associated with a movement disorder. This condition may be especially likely if there is a known history of mental retardation and/or autism in a grandchild. It is likely that psychosomatic medicine physicians do not routinely, in evaluation of dementia cases, inquire about these childhood psychiatric syndromes in the grandchildren of dementia patients. Such cases may benefit from genetic testing of the pedigree to identify full fragile X syndrome and the premutation in other family members. In addition, the premutation state is associated with premature ovarian insufficiency and early menopause. Patients and family members may be screened for this manifestation of the premutation carrier state for fragile X as well.

The inheritance of fragile X syndrome often leads back to a carrier grandparent (more often a grandfather) in the pedigree analysis of an affected child, some of whom have concurrent autism-spectrum psychiatric disorders and significantly impaired psychosocial, occupational, and educational functioning. When genetic testing identifies the grandparent as the source of the genetic mutation that, with genetic amplification, has led to the fragile X syndrome in the grandchild, these patients may experience significant depression related to the guilt of having been "responsible" for their grandchild's genetic illness. This depression over the inheritance of fragile X may be exacerbated by the distress over their own motor impairment; this can be still further exacerbated by these patients' progressive cognitive impairments and/or the depression that may be itself a complication of the FXTAS condition.

These cases offer an opportunity for a multigenerational pedigree analysis, the chance to explore some fascinating family dynamics over the implications of a familial genetic disease, and a new diagnostic possibility in cases of "dementia with a movement disorder." In confirmed cases, connection with the National Fragile X Foundation (http://www.FragileX.org) for background materials and institutional support may be of value for the patients and their families.

Seizure and Venlafaxine Overdose

Venlafaxine is a usually well-tolerated antidepressant with many uses for mood, anxiety, and pain disorders. Although generally safe, it can be dangerous in overdose. Our group had a case of a large venlafaxine overdose associated with seizure activity; seizure risk with venlafaxine is low at usual doses.

> A 22-year-old Hispanic man with a history of major depression and borderline personality disorder had had a previous suicide attempt with an acetaminophen and diphenhydramine overdose combined with alcohol. After recovery from the previous attempt, he was admitted to a psychiatric inpatient unit and treated with venlafaxine 100 mg twice a day for depression. On this regimen, he appeared much less depressed and was discharged. He was given a 30-day supply of medication. Two weeks later, he was readmitted following a venlafaxine overdose. Rescue personnel found him having a tonic-

clonic seizure in his home; he had another tonic-clonic seizure in the emergency department less than 30 minutes later. He was medically stabilized and became fully conscious and was admitted to the hospital. On the second day after admission, he had a dramatic increase in his lactate dehydrogenase (8,542 U/L), aspartate aminotransferase (530 U/L), and creatinine phosphokinase (10,055 U/L). His alanine aminotransferase peaked at 134 U/L on day 6. All these laboratory values had normalized by day 20; venlafaxine was restarted at 37.5 mg daily 2 weeks after the overdose.

◆ **Diagnosis: Axis I—Major Depressive Disorder, Recurrent, Severe Without Psychotic Features, 296.33; Adverse Effects of Medication Not Otherwise Specified, 995.2; Axis II—Borderline Personality Disorder, 301.83**

Psychosomatic medicine psychiatrists evaluating overdose patients who have had access to venlafaxine should consider the possibility of seizure in the occasional patient with an extreme overdose of venlafaxine. Although typically quite safe, venlafaxine in extremely high doses may be associated with more significant symptoms such as seizure; the mechanism for this relationship remains obscure. In addition, large overdoses of venlafaxine may be associated with serotonin syndrome, anticholinergic delirium, and hypertension.

Fahr's Disease With Cognitive Impairment and Paranoia

The clinical evaluation of dementia and psychosis routinely leads to the use of neuroimaging. Especially in patients with a late-life onset of psychosis, the diagnosis of a neurodegenerative condition may explain both the cognitive impairment and the psychotic symptoms.

The patient was a 62-year-old woman with a sensation of "electric shocks" in her chest. Associated with the "shocks" was a conviction that people in her neighborhood were "controlling" her by the use of "electric dials." She became convinced that there were many "microphones" mounted in her home and that her daily activities were being constantly "recorded." In response to these beliefs, she made frequent service calls to the utility company, complaining that "electricity in the air and flickering lights" were causing her various physical symptoms. Her beliefs spread to include a conviction that her bed had become somehow "magnetized" and was then unsafe for sleeping. Her paranoia increased notably following the September 11, 2001, terrorist attacks, because she was concerned for the safety of her daughter, an airline flight attendant. Emergency evaluation of her chest pain revealed normal cardiac studies, and she had no focal neurological signs. Her thyroid-stimulating hormone level was also normal.

She was seen in consultation by psychosomatic medicine because of her paranoid behavior. An additional history of a brief psychiatric admission for paranoid ideation 2 years previously was obtained; however, she had not accepted treatment at that time and was soon released. There was also a distant history of a psychiatric hospitalization, but she would not elaborate on this incident and family members were unable to provide details. On examination, she had floridly paranoid delusions of being controlled by others and being threatened by "electricity," mild psychomotor agitation, and tangentiality. Her MMSE score was 20, with deficits in recall and attention. Affect was nontearful. She was treated with risperidone 0.5 mg orally twice a day. CT scanning revealed bilateral symmetrical basal ganglia calcifications, consistent with Fahr's disease. Following transfer to a psychiatric hospital, she continued to exhibit paranoia about the aforementioned "control" by others, being threatened by "electricity," and being threatened by both neighbors and hospital staff members. Her risperidone was increased to 3 mg at bedtime, and she showed some improvement in her delusion before being discharged.

◆ **Diagnosis: Axis I—Dementia Due to a General Medical Condition, With Behavioral Disturbance, 294.11; Psychotic Disorder Not Otherwise Specified, 298.9**

Fahr's disease includes basal ganglia calcifications associated with neuropsychiatric symptoms, including movement disorders, stroke-like events, psychosis, mood disorders, and dementia. A substantial percentage of patients have no motor symptoms and present with purely psychiatric symptoms. There may be systemic disorders of calcium metabolism associated with the basal ganglia calcification, but many cases are idiopathic. Because of the possibility of movement disorders in Fahr's disease, it seems especially prudent to use atypical antipsychotic agents when treating psychotic symptoms in these patients.

Seizure and Delirium Associated With Clozapine

Clozapine is a major advance in the treatment of otherwise unresponsive schizophrenia. However, it is rife with systemic side effects based on its multiple receptor actions. The psychosomatic medicine physician is occasionally confronted with the management of schizophrenic patients who have (paradoxically) heretofore had a good clinical response to clozapine in terms of psychotic symptoms but who then have significant systemic side effects from clozapine that render its further use problematic or even dangerous.

> The patient was a 64-year-old white man with a long history of paranoid schizophrenia, which in recent years had been complicated by mood symptoms. He had been treated over the years with many combinations of psychotropic medications, numerous psychiatric hospitalizations, and ECT. Prior to his decompensation and hospital admission, he had been doing relatively well on the combination of clozapine 700 mg daily, benztropine 1 mg daily, paroxetine 40 mg daily, clonazepam 1 mg daily, and perphenazine 48 mg daily. His only recent medication change was a decrease in his daily clozapine dosage from 800 mg to 700 mg. He was living under supervision of a legal conservator in a board and care facility, where he was compliant with his medications and had shown no behavioral deterioration over a long period of time. However, he then experienced several episodes of altered level of consciousness, loss of postural tone, and seizure activity. He had no previous history of seizure disorder.
>
> On admission, he had renal insufficiency with blood urea nitrogen and creatinine levels of 56 mg/dL and 2.6 mg/dL, respectively. Sodium and potassium levels were unremarkable; complete blood cell count showed increased white blood cells and mild anemia. Creatinine phosphokinase was elevated at 2,040 U/L. On examination, he was afebrile with stable vital signs. He was restrained in a Posey belt. He had largely nonsensical speech. He was neither tremulous nor rigid. He had a vacant and vacuous gaze, no suicidal or homicidal ideations, and an MMSE score of 0. He was diagnosed with schizophrenia, delirium, and rule out dementia. Because it was imperative to minimize delirium-promoting agents to control his delirium, paroxetine, clonazepam, benztropine, perphenazine and clozapine were held. Electroencephalograms and neurology consultation were ordered to rule out clozapine-associated seizure disorder.
>
> Two days later, he was somewhat improved, with an MMSE score of 9. He was more able to converse and had more organized thought processes. A neurology consultation confirmed a recent seizure. By

this time his creatinine phosphokinase, blood urea nitrogen, and creatinine levels had normalized. MRI showed diffuse cortical atrophy. His electroencephalogram showed temporal spikes and generalized slowing. For seizure control, he was treated with carbamazepine 400 mg daily. In light of the seizure disorder confirmed by neurology, it was felt to be unsafe to continue clozapine, and he was now started on olanzapine 10 mg daily.

By hospital day 12, his MMSE score had improved to 21. As he became more verbal and organized, he voiced paranoid delusions of others "trying to get" him, visions of "the Devil" and auditory hallucinations telling him to hurt himself. His olanzapine was gradually up-tapered in an attempt to control his psychosis; his dosage by the end of the hospital stay was 35 mg daily. For further control of his seizure activity, he was also started on dilantin 300 mg daily. His MMSE scores further improved to 27 by hospital day 19 and to 29 by hospital day 31. Although his delirium and seizures had cleared and he was now on stable seizure prophylaxis, he continued to experience disturbing command auditory hallucinations. Once he was medically cleared, he was then transferred to an inpatient psychiatric facility for continued care.

◆ **Diagnosis: Axis I—Schizophrenia, Paranoid Type, 295.30; Delirium, 293.0; Adverse Side Effects of Medication Not Otherwise Specified, 995.2**

This case illustrates, in graphic form, a dilemma. On the one hand, this was a severely impaired schizophrenic patient who had been stabilized on clozapine (in addition to other medications) and who was able, for a time, to maintain a reasonable level of social function under supervision. However, he experienced a seizure and delirium. For all of its other obvious benefits, clozapine is known to decrease the seizure threshold, to increase the risk of syncope (via its α-adrenergic effects), and to decrease cognitive function (via its anticholinergic effects). Discontinuing clozapine (and other psychopharmacologic agents with potential to exacerbate delirium) and managing his seizure disorder were associated with clearing of his delirium and recovery of his cognitive function; in addition, he had no further episodes of loss of consciousness or falls. However, he remained paranoid and in need of psychiatric hospitalization.

In the acute medical center setting, it was necessary to discontinue clozapine in order to fully evaluate and manage delirium and to address the possibility of a seizure disorder as contributing to this patient's acute presentation. Should he remain profoundly psychotic, it may be possible, under "cover" of continued seizure prophylaxis and with due caution, to carefully rechallenge him with clozapine under controlled conditions. Psychosomatic medicine physicians must be willing to address the possibility of clozapine side effects in the acute presentation of delirium in clozapine patients, leaving the background psychotic illness for later management after the delirium aspects of the case have been managed.

Head Trauma and Acute Stress Disorder

When practicing psychosomatic medicine in a medical center, particularly a trauma center, one will frequently encounter TBI patients (Bryant and Harvey 1998; Fann et al. 2004; Rao and Lyketsos 2000). Indeed, psychosomatic medicine psychiatrists practicing in Department of Defense and Department of Veterans Affairs facilities are particularly likely to encounter TBI patients among active-duty military personnel and veterans. The TBI patients often present with a "telescoping" series of psychiatric symptoms, depending on the proximity of their clinical presentation to the serious injury producing TBI. Symptoms often change significantly over time as the patient recovers. Notably, traumatic memories of the major events leading to TBI may not be present initially, when cognitive function is decreased, because acute amnesia may interfere with the memories of the event that resulted in the physical trauma.

Psychopharmacological approaches may need modification over time as different symptom profiles emerge and "replace" each other. In addition, the psychotherapy approaches to these patients may need to be modified to a "here-and-now" approach, because often these patients must confront not only psychological adaptation to physical injuries but also the loss of friends and family members who may have perished in the same traumatic event.

Case 1

The patient was a 20-year-old victim of a motor vehicle accident. He presented initially with confusion, altered sleep-wake cycle, episodes of agitated behavior, and an inability to work with physical therapists on the trauma service. His initial MMSE score was 20, with deficits in memory, concentration, and orientation. He was amnestic for the accident and the events immediately prior to it. He showed mild cognitive disorganization and was slow to learn therapy activities. He was given a low dose of risperidone, 0.5 mg orally at bedtime.

Over several days, his confusion resolved and his MMSE score improved. However, at this point he began to acquire memories of the accident. His sleep, initially improved on risperidone, now became fragmented and punctuated by vivid nightmares of the event. His mood became anxiously depressed. During the day, he developed flashbacks and avoided newspaper and television accounts of other vehicular accidents, because these provoked further traumatic memories. To improve sleep and to address the emergent mood and anxiety symptoms, mirtazapine 15 mg orally at bedtime was added to his continued low dose of risperidone. After several more days, his sleep pattern had normalized, the nightmares had significantly decreased, and the flashbacks and avoidance behaviors were largely resolved.

♦ **Diagnosis: Axis I—Acute Stress Disorder, 308.3; Delirium, 293.0**

This case illustrates that TBI patients may initially present with mildly impaired cognition on examination, which correlates with poor memory of details of the traumatic event. Empirical treatment of the cognitive and sleep complaints may be associated with functional improvement. However, as cognitive function improves, memories of the inciting trauma may emerge. Patients may then benefit from specific treatment with a sedative and/or an antidepressant to address acute stress disorder symptoms. Because of the delay in the presentation of acute stress disorder, this can be thought of as "tardive onset acute stress disorder."

Case 2

The second patient was a 19-year-old man. He was the driver of a vehicle in which two of his passengers (both were his close friends) were killed. Although the legal aspects of the case were not adjudicated during our care of this man, the initial legal response was to charge him with culpability in the accident, and there was a consideration of formal criminal charges of negligent homicide. His family, recently arrived from the Middle East, were dually devastated; first they were concerned that their young adult son (a university honor student with plans to become a pharmacist) was now hospitalized with severe orthopedic injuries, and second they had a large degree of shame and guilt that his driving was the putative cause of the deaths of two other young men.

Psychosomatic medicine was consulted. The patient was experiencing insomnia, vivid flashbacks of the accident, the bloody accident scene, images of his friends dying at the scene, and penetrating loud noises of vehicles crashing. Although not actively suicidal, he had enormous amounts of survivor guilt, stating that he wished he could have died rather than his friends. In addition, he believed that his plans to further his education, for which his family had made significant sacrifices, were now shattered. All these concerns were potentiated by the expectation that he would be held legally liable for his friends' deaths.

He was treated with mirtazapine 15 mg at bedtime to offer sedation and to treat his mood symptoms. After several days, his sleep and nightmares improved. He remained depressed and deeply regretful over his friends' deaths but was more able to work on his rehabilitation tasks and to work on the profound changes in his life.

◆ **Diagnosis: Axis I—Acute Stress Disorder, 308.3**

This case, in addition to the dramatic and tragic life-altering story it represents, illustrates a classic case of acute stress disorder with significant "survivor guilt." This is obviously accentuated by the very real prospect of facing civil or even criminal legal consequences for any culpability. Because of the likelihood of traumatic reexperiencing of the accident in the posthospitalization period, early symptomatic treatment started in hospital and close outpatient follow-up are most recommended.

Case 3

The third patient was a 36-year-old white man with a history of alcohol and drug abuse who was struck by a train. He experienced multiple traumas including a basilar skull fracture. CT of the head revealed pneumocranium and left lenticular nucleus infarct. He experienced significant cognitive deficits (e.g., he was unable to learn that his mother had died early in his hospitalization, despite having been told this sad news numerous times) and dysphoric mood. On initial psychosomatic medicine consultation (2 months after admission) he had an MMSE score of 18, irritably dysphoric affect, and concrete but reasonably coherent thought processes.

Because he had persistent cognitive deficits 2 months after a TBI, he was started on donepezil 5 mg/day. In 10 days, his MMSE score was 23, and risperidone and venlafaxine were added; these dosages were gradually adjusted to 2 mg at bedtime and 150 mg in the morning, respectively. Over the next month, his irritably dysphoric affect improved notably, and his MMSE improved still further to 28. With this level of improved cognition and mood, he was finally able to understand the specifics of his accident. Notably, he was also now able to learn of his mother's death and was able to process her loss reasonably well.

◆ **Diagnosis: Axis I—Polysubstance Dependence, 304.80; Depressive Disorder Not Otherwise Specified, 311; Cognitive Disorder Not Otherwise Specified, 294.9**

Case 4

The fourth patient was a 35-year-old white man with a history of polysubstance abuse and antisocial behavior (having just been released from prison for a drug sentence) who was injured in a motor vehicle accident: he was found by emergency rescue personnel unconscious and 30 feet from his demolished vehicle. He experienced multiple traumas and a period of hypothermia. An initial CT scan of the head was negative for fracture or hemorrhage. He received initial surgical management of his thoracic and abdominal injuries with exploratory laparotomy with splenectomy, liver laceration repair, and bilateral chest tube placement. He subsequently needed surgical drainage of several fluid collections and treatment for infections.

He was seen by the psychosomatic medicine service on hospital day 11, at which time examination revealed motor agitation. He was unable to cooperate with the balance of the examination. Repeated neuroimaging revealed bilateral subdural fluid collections. Electroencephalograms revealed bilateral slowing. He was started on risperidone for agitation; the dosage was titrated to 6 mg/day in divided doses. He then had decreased agitation and increasing periods of wakefulness and responsiveness. During his fifth week of hospitalization, his mental status improved to a condition of limited spontaneous and dysarthric speech; perplexed, nontearful affect; poor ability to initiate purposeful behavior; and poor memory and attention. His MMSE score was now 4. Because of his persistent cognitive impairment, he was started on donepezil 5 mg in the morning (later increased to 10 mg in the morning) and amantadine 200 mg twice a day. His delirium improved, and his MMSE score improved to 17 within 2 more weeks.

However, as his cognition improved (albeit with significant residual deficits), his behavior became more agitated and aggressive. He did not appear to be responding to internal stimuli and did not verbalize paranoid delusions. Risperidone was discontinued, and valproate 500 mg twice a day was started. He then became less aggressive and irritable. In the eighth week of hospitalization, his MMSE score rose to 20, and he could finally answer questions of his personal history and orient more accurately to time and place, although he remained amnestic for any substantive details of the accident. At an MMSE score of 24, he was noted to have mildly depressed mood and poor concentration; venlafaxine extended release, 75 mg in the morning, was added. After approximately 30 days of treatment, amantadine and donepezil were both tapered and discontinued. His final MMSE score was 28, and he was discharged in stable condition, still receiving venlafaxine and valproate.

◆ **Diagnosis: Axis I—Polysubstance Dependence, 304.80; Cognitive Disorder Not Otherwise Specified, 294.9; Depressive Disorder Not Otherwise Specified, 311; Axis II—Antisocial Traits**

These last two cases illustrate persistent cognitive deficits associated with symptoms of a mood disorder. Psychopharmacological treatment of mental status changes may be helpful in optimizing psychiatric function for the challenging tasks of rehabilitation of the physical and psychological trauma, as well as adaptation to new and often profound limitations in psychosocial function. The close connection between mood state and cognitive status is also important to recognize; the tendency to see different realms of psychological function in "parallel channels" fails to recognize that optimal cognitive function depends on a relatively intact mood state and freedom from agitation and psychosis.

Prion Disease

Although rare and uniformly devastating, prion disease should be considered as a possibility in certain dementia presentations. We evaluated a case of prion disease in a patient with an initially ambiguous presentation.

The patient was a 70-year-old white man with an unremarkable medical history. He was admitted to the neurology service with new-onset tremors. While being evaluated by the neurology service, he was described as being "uncooperative," and consultation was requested to "rule out conversion disorder." According to family members, he had been doing well until relatively recently, when he had begun to act "confused" and to have abnormal movements. This had led to his admission to the hospital.

On examination, he had notable tremors and athetoid movements of the extremities. He was alert but had mildly dysarthric speech. His cognitive examination was impaired, with an MMSE score of 16. CT of the head revealed atrophy; a subsequent electro-encephalogram revealed triphasic waves classic for Creutzfeldt-Jakob disease. Upon further inquiry, no exposure to tissue grafts or other potentially prion-contaminated biological material could be ascertained. He had an unfortunately progressive downhill course, with increasing cognitive impairment, leading to his death 2 months later.

♦ **Diagnosis: Axis I—Dementia Due to a General Medical Condition, 294.10**

Such cases, with an inherently grim prognosis and little room for clinical intervention, are fortunately rare. Remarkable about this presentation was the initial request for consultation based on concern for "conversion disorder." Upon our evaluation and determination of impaired cognition, the workup progressed from "rule out conversion disorder" to "dementia with a movement disorder." The concurrence of dementia with movement disorder symptoms should lead the clinician to consider the possibility of prion disease, especially in cases with rapid progression of simultaneous movement disorder and cognitive impairment.

Poststroke Depression, Apathy, and Modafinil

Depressed states occurring in the first year after a stroke may be classified as poststroke depression. Patients with this diagnosis may or may not have had a history of previous mood disorders. When these patients present with depressed states (especially if there is a prominent component of apathy), their activity and participation in important rehabilitative activities may be seriously compromised. Thus, early clinical intervention to improve the mood state may be important to facilitate their recovery.

The patient was a 70-year-old white woman with a history of bipolar disorder, for which she had been treated with maintenance lithium carbonate, 600 mg daily. She had not had significant mood episodes for many years. She was also treated with levothyroxine for hypothyroidism and had a history of hyperlipidemia and hypertension. She subacutely developed increasingly worsening headaches and eventually developed a period of loss of consciousness. She was emergently evaluated with CT and found to have a ruptured aneurysm of the basilar artery. She underwent an endovascular coiling procedure to treat the aneurysm; she was subsequently found to also have a frontal lobe hydrocephalus, which was treated with a right frontal ventriculostomy. Postoperatively, she gradually regained consciousness but could not follow verbal directions. After a period of approximately 3 weeks following neurosurgery, she was transferred to the rehabilitation service.

While on the rehabilitation service, she was described by physicians and staff to be "apathetic and lethargic" and not participating actively in the various therapy activities. There were no symptoms of anxiety, mania/hypomania, or psychosis. She was seen by the psychosomatic medicine service for evaluation of poststroke depression. Upon evaluation, she was alert but disoriented in three spheres, with flat affect and sparse spontaneous speech. She was unable to complete any of the items of the MMSE. She denied suicidality and hallucinations. Lithium (which had been maintained at the usual dosage throughout this time) was discontinued and, in view of the patient's extremely depressed and apathetic appearance, modafinil 100 mg daily was started. Within 3 days she was notably more animated and verbal. Ten days after beginning modafinil, she was now able to score 21 on the MMSE. Upon recovery, she was able to actively participate in therapy activities and made rapid progress. She was able to be discharged to her home in stable condition (still receiving modafinil), having achieved all of her needed rehabilitation goals.

When she was seen in psychiatry clinic 2 weeks after discharge from the rehabilitation service, her mood symptoms continued to show improvement. She had no further apathy and no neurovegetative symptoms. She had normal levels of spontaneous speech. She had no symptoms suggesting hypomania or mania. At home, she continued to exhibit memory problems in daily activities (requiring family support) but was able to accomplish most of her activities of daily living. A repeat MMSE was given, on which her score was 20. She was maintained on modafinil.

◆ **Diagnosis: Axis I—Mood Disorder Due to a General Medical Condition, With Depressive Features, 293.83;**

Bipolar Disorder Not Otherwise Specified (by History), 296.80; Rule Out Vascular Dementia, With Depressed Mood, 290.43

This patient had a history of compensated bipolar disorder on lithium maintenance; she had gone several years without a significant mood episode. She then presented with an acute stroke. Neurosurgical interventions were associated with complications and a long period of medical recovery. Poststroke, she had a depressive episode with a significant apathy component. Treatment with the "wakefulness promoter" modafinil was associated with a prompt and ultimately sustained response. As her mood state improved, she was able to exhibit improved cognitive function, albeit still in the range of cognitive impairment.

Conventional antidepressants, such as selective serotonin reuptake inhibitors and tricyclic antidepressants, have been used for poststroke depression with generally favorable results. In this case, because the patient's initial presentation was notable for profound apathy, modafinil was chosen for a more immediate effect, specifically on the apathy component of the case. Modafinil may be ultimately preferable to conventional psychostimulants in such cases by virtue of less risk for hypertension, insomnia, anxiety, and tachycardia than the conventional agents. The risk of medication-induced hypomania or mania, especially in a patient with a history of bipolar disorder, warrants due caution and close clinical monitoring throughout the period of modafinil therapy.

Because strokes will typically occur in patients with multiple vascular risk factors (hypertension, diabetes mellitus, hypercholesterolemia, and smoking), poststroke mood disorder patients are, by definition, at risk for vascular dementia as well. In particular, when poststroke patients exhibit aphasia, it may be difficult to ascertain whether the cognitive impairment (often newly discovered) is itself a consequence of the stroke, a functional cognitive consequence of poststroke depression (which may improve with treatment), or perhaps a preexisting cognitive impairment that had previously eluded clinical attention. Following the patient carefully over the first poststroke year and monitoring the cognitive status along with the mood status may allow for some clarification of these points.

Psychosomatic medicine psychiatrists should be alert to post-stroke depression in the stroke patients whom they treat (Robinson 1997). Thoughtful application of psychopharmacological principles in these cases may allow for improved mood, a greater capacity for productive use of poststroke rehabilitation activities, and better functional status.

Poststroke Mania

Although likely far less common than poststroke depression, post-stroke mood disorders on the bipolar spectrum may occur, typically in patients with no history of bipolar disorders (Starkstein et al. 1991). The behavioral manifestations of poststroke bipolar disorder may be extremely disruptive to the rehabilitative care these patients need to optimize their recovery and functional improvement. Clinical intervention with psychotropic medication is often a crucial part of treatment. Psychosomatic medicine physicians treating post-stroke patients should keep this diagnostic possibility in mind.

> The patient was a 70-year-old man with a negative psychiatric history. He had an acute loss of consciousness and was brought to the emergency department. Upon examination he had confusion, left-sided hemiplegia, and neglect of the left visual space. CT revealed a large infarct of the right middle cerebral artery with surrounding edema. He was treated and stabilized and then transferred to physical medicine and rehabilitation for poststroke rehabilitation. He continued to have hemiparesis and neglect of the left visual space.
>
> While on the physical medicine and rehabilitation service, he was noted to have minimal need for sleep, to be irritable and distractible from rehabilitation tasks, and to be speaking rapidly and in a pressured fashion. A psychosomatic medicine consultation was obtained. On examination he was expansive, irritable, and distractible. He spoke rapidly and was difficult to interrupt. He was disoriented for place and time and scored 7 on his initial MMSE. Poststroke mood disorder, bipolar type, with a hypomanic episode was diagnosed. He was started on olanzapine, 2.5 mg in the morning and 5 mg at bedtime. Within 3 days, he had a much improved sleep pattern and was no longer irritable. His speech slowed considerably and was no longer pressured. He was able to orient much more accurately and could demonstrate improved cognitive function; his later MMSE score was 23. During this period, importantly, he was much

more focused on rehabilitation tasks and was increasingly able to manage more of his activities of daily living with less supervision.

◆ **Diagnosis: Axis I—Mood Disorder Due to a General Medical Condition, With Manic Features, 293.83; Vascular Dementia, With Delusions, 290.42**

This was a case of poststroke bipolar disorder. The classic laterality of poststroke depression is with a left-sided lesion. Although much less common than poststroke depression, poststroke bipolar disorder and poststroke psychotic disorder are typically associated with a right-sided lesion. Because of his manic symptoms, the patient's behavior on the rehabilitation service was quite disruptive, and his progress on cognitive rehabilitation had been minimal, to the point where the physical medicine and rehabilitation service was actively considering curtailing the rehabilitation intervention and discharging him to a skilled nursing facility. After treatment with an atypical antipsychotic agent, his sleep pattern quickly returned to normal, his mood stabilized, and his attention and cognitive function improved dramatically. His final MMSE score of 23 was felt to represent mild residual vascular dementia; donepezil was then started and was well tolerated. His mood and cognitive function remained in their improved condition for the balance of the hospitalization. He was eventually able to be discharged to his family with geriatric psychiatry clinical follow-up.

This case illustrates two important points in the management of poststroke patients. First, poststroke patients should be routinely screened for depression, mania, and psychotic disorders. Once treated, this man's condition and capacity to participate in rehabilitation improved markedly. Second, this case demonstrates an intimate connection between mood and cognition. Simple cognitive testing without assessment of the mood state in an integrated fashion could have led to the false impression that the case was primarily one of poststroke dementia. However, rapid identification of the mood disorder and prompt treatment with a mood stabilizer was associated secondarily with a precipitous increase in cognitive function, a rate of cognitive improvement that would not be expected with simple healing of the vascular lesion.

Corticosteroid-Associated Mania

A 45-year-old female patient with multiple sclerosis with a chronically relapsing/remitting course was admitted to the medical center with an exacerbation of her motor symptoms. She was given a short course of corticosteroids (prednisone), which was quickly tapered from the maximum dosage of 100 mg/day. Within days of the corticosteroid course beginning, she developed decreased need for sleep, racing thoughts, pressured speech, irritable affect, and grandiosity. She had no prior history of bipolar disorder.

She was treated with olanzapine 10 mg at bedtime and 5 mg orally every 6 hours as needed for agitation. Within days of starting the olanzapine, she had an improved sleep pattern, less irritability, normal speech, and relief from racing thoughts. The olanzapine was continued for several days after the end of the brief course of prednisone, at which time it was tapered and discontinued.

◆ **Diagnosis: Axis I—Mood Disorder Due to a General Medical Condition, With Manic Features, 293.83**

This case illustrates the presentation of corticosteroid-associated mania. This risk is greater if the daily dosage of corticosteroid is 40 mg of prednisone and may be more likely if dosages are changed rapidly from baseline, as in the "burst" therapy typically used for exacerbations of multiple sclerosis. In this particular case, the psychiatrist must consider the possibility of a mood disorder due to the multiple sclerosis itself; the presentation of mood symptoms soon after the use of corticosteroids makes this possibility less likely, because mood disorder (bipolar type) associated with multiple sclerosis, rather than its treatment, would more likely be associated with the change in motor symptoms, not the corticosteroid dosing. Of course, this relationship is by nature somewhat imprecise, and mood disorder, bipolar type, associated with underlying multiple sclerosis should be considered as the diagnosis if there are several episodes of mood elevation apparently unrelated to medications for multiple sclerosis per se.

Manic episodes directly attributable to systemic or CNS conditions or systemic medications are much more infrequent than depressive episodes. Other examples of conditions associated with manic episodes include traumatic brain injury, cerebrovascular accident (a higher risk with right-sided lesions has been described), CNS tumors, and giant cell arteritis. Because of their common use for a variety of inflammatory and degenerative conditions, corticosteroids represent one of the more important causes of medication-induced mania. The paradox in this sort of condition is that although the corticosteroids typically improve the underlying neurological condition temporarily (e.g., in the treatment of the multiple sclerosis exacerbation), their psychiatric side effects (in this case, mood disturbance) may be additive to the already established mood disorder associated with the underlying systemic condition. Regarding pharmacological treatment for mania associated with systemic illness and/or medications, treatment paradigms need to be modified.

Thoughtful and informed empiricism remains the mainstay of interventions. Brief treatment of manic episodes with atypical antipsychotics offers the best hope for a prompt response, and there may be little need for maintenance treatment as long as the putative precipitant (high-dose corticosteroid in this case) is discontinued after the systemic symptoms have improved. Distinguishing medication-associated mania from either classic bipolar disorder (that just "happens" to be present in a patient with an unrelated systemic illness) or mood disorder, bipolar type, due to a general medical condition (as a physiological consequence of the underlying systemic illness) remains a true test of the psychiatrist's experience, clinical judgment, and capacity for inferential thinking.

To be most convincing as a case of "pure" medication-induced mood or psychotic disorder, the psychiatric episode should only be present in the context of the medication being given, should not be present premorbidly, and should only recur in the context of reexposure to the implicated medication. In a condition such as multiple sclerosis, there is the possibility that the underlying medical condition itself is responsible for the mood/psychotic exacerbation. In such a case, it is most convincing if the mood/psychotic symptoms proceed "in concert with" other physical findings (e.g., increased motor symptoms in multiple sclerosis correlating temporally with psychiatric symptoms) *before* exposure to an immunosuppressant.

Often, these distinctions are initially subtle and require a period of longitudinal observation of the patient's experience and a clinical willingness to treat episodes in advance of satisfying diagnostic precision.

Retrograde Amnesia

Dementing disorders are characterized by retrograde and/or anterograde amnesia, evidence of other cognitive impairment, and a full
level of consciousness. In the general hospital, where the psychosomatic medicine specialist sees the bulk of patients, dementia patients
may be physically disruptive and dangerous, quietly and compliantly
confused, or a combination of these. Often, a significant degree of
retrograde amnesia may "propel" the patient back in time to a period
that is more familiar and somewhat comforting. Memory is often lost
in inverse order of acquisition but with some internal consistency. Interviewer insertion of accurate contemporary information can dis-
rupt this sense of comfort and lead to ironic consequences.

Case 1: The War With Guatemala

The patient was a 75-year-old African American man with a history
of progressive cognitive deficits to the point that he was unable to
care for himself at home. Family members were unable to provide
constant supervision. Because of some disorganized behavior, he
was admitted to the hospital for evaluation and placement. On interview, he was pleasant and cooperative but perplexed. He could
not say why he was in a hospital or even whether he was in a hospital,
saying he was "just not sure." He answered questions diligently and
sincerely, without irritability.

His degree of retrograde amnesia, however, was remarkable.
When asked the current year (factually 1990), he quickly replied
"1943." When asked as a follow-up question about the current
events, he replied "the war, of course." When asked who the enemy
of the United States was in the war, he replied "Guatemala." When
interviewed the next day, he continued to orient to "1943" and "the
war with Guatemala."

On a subsequent interview, he said, yet again, that it was "1943."
When asked a third time about current events, he replied, "the war, of
course. We are still fighting." When asked about the enemy, he now
said "not Guatemala any more. We kicked their butts off yesterday!"

◆ **Diagnosis: Axis I—Dementia of the Alzheimer's Type, 294.10**

Case 2:"Eisenhower, You Fool!"

Another dementia patient with severe retrograde amnesia presented
with more irritability. This man was a 75-year-old white man, also
admitted in 1990, following agitated behavior and assaultiveness at

his nursing home. He had had a several-year history of cognitive impairment associated with aggressive acting-out behavior. Because his skilled nursing facility could no longer manage him, he was admitted for evaluation and placement.

When approached for an initial interview, he glowered suspiciously before gruffly demanding, "Who the hell are you?" He was minimally cooperative, stating that he did not "see the need for all these silly questions. I'm just fine!" At the orientation component of the mental status examination, his situation became clear.

"What year is it now?" he was asked, to which he replied, "What do you mean what year is it? Everyone knows what the year is!" Following persistent questioning, he finally bellowed "1955. Everyone knows it's 1955!" The conversation continued thus:

CLINICIAN: Are you sure?

PATIENT: Of course I'm sure!

CLINICIAN: Then, I am sure you can tell me who the president of the U.S. is now, can't you?

PATIENT: The president, of course! President Eisenhower, you fool!

CLINICIAN: Then who is this man, president [George H.W.] Bush we hear about?

PATIENT: Bush? Bush? Never heard of him. Probably some half-witted politician!

CLINICIAN: Do you like baseball?"

PATIENT: Of course, everyone likes baseball!

CLINICIAN: Then you must have a favorite baseball team.

PATIENT: The Brooklyn Dodgers. They just won the World Series, you know!

Allowing for the challenges in communication caused by his irritability, this man was living as though in 1955. Notably, the historical events he recalled were accurate, at least from a frame of reference of 1955. Gentle attempts to reorient him were quickly rebuffed, and he spent his entire 1990 hospitalization firmly rooted in 1955.

◆ **Diagnosis: Axis I—Dementia of the Alzheimer's Type, 294.10**

The degree of retrograde amnesia in severe dementia may be quite profound, as in these cases. In severely impaired patients who have relatively preserved verbal and language function, the experience of being with them can create a sense of a being in a "time warp." It is helpful to have at least some rudimentary knowledge of the historical period to which the patient has regressed. It is likely that the perplexity and/or agitation experienced by these patients have their genesis in a sense of not fitting into the current time reality, and they may find comfort in their retrograde amnesiac alternative reality. Confrontation and attempts to reorient in terms of time to the current reality may not be fruitful; empathic attempts to understand where and when the patient finds him- or herself may lead to a greater understanding of the patient's experience.

References

American Psychiatric Association: Diagnostic and Statistical Manual of Mental Disorders, 4th Edition, Text Revision. Washington, DC, American Psychiatric Association, 2000

Applebaum PS, Grisso T: Assessing patients' capacity to consent to treatment. N Engl J Med 319:1635–1638, 1988

Asperger H: Die "Autistischen psychopathen" im Kindesalter. Arch Psychiatr Nervenk 117:76–136, 1944

Baron-Cohen S, Jolliffe T, Mortimore C, et al: Another advanced test of theory of mind: evidence from very high functioning adults with autism or Asperger syndrome. J Child Psychol Psychiatry 38:813–822, 1997

Baron-Cohen S, Wheelwright S, Robinson J, et al: The adult Asperger Assessment (AAA): a diagnostic method. J Autism Dev Disord 35:807–819, 2005

Bonelli RM, Cummings JC: Frontal-subcortical dementias. Neurologist 14:100–107, 2008

Bryant RA, Harvey AG: Relationship between acute stress disorder and post-traumatic stress disorder following mild traumatic brain injury. Am J Psychiatry 155:625–629, 1998

Duffy JD, Campbell JJ 3rd: The regional prefrontal syndromes: a theoretical and clinical overview. J Neuropsychiatry Clin Neurosci 6:379–387, 1994

Fann JR, Burington B, Leonetti A, et al: Psychiatric illness following traumatic brain injury in an adult health maintenance organization population. Arch Gen Psychiatry 61:53–61, 2004

Folstein MF, Folstein SE, McHugh PR: "Mini-Mental State": a practical method for grading the cognitive state of patients for the clinician. J Psychiatr Res 12:189–198, 1975

Hagerman PJ, Hagerman RJ: Fragile X-associated tremor/ataxia syndrome (FXTAS). Ment Retard Dev Disabil Res Rev 10:25–30, 2004

Jacquemont S, Hagerman RJ, Leehey M, et al: Fragile X premutation tremor/ataxia syndrome: molecular, clinical, and neuroimaging correlates. Am J Hum Genet 72:869–878, 2003

Marsh L: Neuropsychiatric aspects of Parkinson's disease. Psychosomatics 41:15–23, 2000

Physicians' Desk Reference. Montvale, NJ, Thompson PDR, 2007

Rao V, Lyketsos C: Neuropsychiatric sequelae of traumatic brain injury. Psychosomatics 41:93–105, 2000

Robinson RG: Neuropsychiatric consequences of stroke. Annu Rev Med 48:217–229, 1997

Rosenblatt A, Leroi I: Neuropsychiatry of Huntington's disease and other basal ganglia disorders. Psychosomatics 41:24–30, 2000

Starkstein SE, Federoff P, Berthier ML, et al: Manic-depressive and pure manic states after brain lesions. Biol Psychiatry 29:149–158, 1991

Wing L: Asperger's syndrome: a clinical account. Psychol Med 11:115–129, 1981

15

OBSTETRICS AND GYNECOLOGY AND PEDIATRICS

Obstetrics and gynecology and pediatrics are areas sometimes associated with emotionally laden cases for psychosomatic medicine consultants. Disruptive clinical events in these two specialties may lead to a need for prompt, thoughtful, and creative consultation. Dealing with hospital staff countertransference may be particularly important in these cases.

Denied Pregnancy

The patient was a 21-year-old single white female medical technician. She reported for her usual night shift on a medical ward. Midway through the shift, she left her job station and went into an unoccupied patient room. There, she precipitously and without assistance delivered a viable full-term male infant. She wrapped the newborn in a blanket and put him on a patient bed and then proceeded to clean herself of the products of childbirth in the bathroom. A ward nurse heard the newborn crying and came to assist him, coincidentally discovering the patient. She was admitted to the obstetric service, and the child was admitted to the nursery.

When seen in psychosomatic medicine consultation the next morning, the patient denied any psychiatric history or any current mood, anxiety, psychotic, or cognitive symptoms. She was unmarried, and her family of origin lived in another part of the country. She had an ongoing relationship with a boyfriend who was not the father of the newborn. She denied knowing she had been pregnant, attributing her pregnancy symptoms to gradual weight gain from "overeating and not exercising." She stated she had no conscious knowledge she was pregnant until she had gone into labor the night before, when "it hit me all at once."

The patient was from a strict and conservative religious background in which single motherhood was highly frowned upon. It was psychologically unacceptable for her to be an "unwed mother," so she denied the pregnancy. She did not deny the pregnancy in a psychotic way, for example, attributing the pregnancy symptoms to psychotic causes. When confronted on the reality of the newborn's existence, she readily embraced the maternal role and unequivocally wanted to keep and raise the newborn. She received regular counseling and social supports. Over several months of close follow-up by Child Protective Services representatives, she adapted well to parenthood and had no other episodes of psychiatric symptoms.

◆ **Diagnosis: Axis I—Psychological Factors Affecting Physical Condition, 316; Adjustment Disorder Unspecified, 309.9**

This case illustrates the disruption that can result from a denied pregnancy, especially when the patient is herself a hospital employee. Obviously, the precipitous birth in the middle of a shift is an enormous disruption; the more so when the pregnancy was denied all along. The ability of this patient's working colleagues to rally around and assist her after she delivered was remarkable; perhaps the support given her in the workplace was a key factor in her ability to successfully bond to and raise the child.

Psychosomatic medicine psychiatrists may be called on to evaluate patients with denied pregnancy in the context of the obstetric service, when these women present suddenly in labor and are able to "deny" their condition no more. The adjustments to motherhood and its related social roles may be profoundly difficult in such a case; certainly, the expectation is that there will be a large need for social support agencies for these women.

Shaken—Not Infected—Baby

The patient was a 5-month-old girl transferred to the Pediatric Intensive Care Unit (PICU) at a tertiary care teaching center from an outlying rural hospital with presumed disseminated meningococcal disease. The child had been in the care of her mother's boyfriend of 3 months while the mother worked the graveyard shift as a shelf-stocker at Wal-Mart. When the child's mother returned the next morning, she found her daughter listless, barely arousable, and uninterested in feeding, with dusky pallor and prominent contusions and petechiae over her limbs, trunk, and scalp. The boyfriend reported that the infant had slept through the night after taking her 10:00 P.M. bottle without complaint.

The patient's mother called 911, and the emergency medicine technicians rushed her to the local hospital for stabilization in preparation for transfer. Because she appeared to be seizing, she was loaded with anticonvulsants and intubated. She also underwent an infectious disease workup that included lumbar puncture, venipuncture, and bladder tap as well as prophylactic broad-spectrum antibiotics.

At the receiving medical center, she was initially treated as though she had an infectious diathesis for her signs and symptoms. Additional social history revealed that the child's mother and her boyfriend had only lived together for the past 6 weeks and that the boyfriend was easily angered by the normal fussing of the infant, although no one had seen him try to harm the child.

The baby was the result of an uncomplicated, full-term pregnancy, with a birth weight of 3,700 grams (8.1 lb). She had several weeks earlier appeared to sustain an injury when the boyfriend "accidentally" jammed the front passenger seat backwards, catching her left leg between his seat and her car seat. Although she had been crying at the time and the boyfriend was obviously agitated when he shoved his seat backwards, her mother focused on comforting the child rather than confronting her partner about his aggressive act. After initially squalling, the child calmed with acetaminophen for pain.

Over the days following admission, all cultures came back negative, and the patient was stabilized without further extension or exacerbation of the prominent skin findings. An alert intern noted that the bruises on the infant's upper arms corresponded to an adult's fingerprints. Given the inconclusive infectious disease workup and growing doubts about the reliability of the boyfriend's story, the PICU team decided to pursue a trauma survey. A magnetic resonance imaging scan revealed bilateral intracranial hemorrhages and retinal hemorrhages consistent with a shaking injury. Moreover, long-bone X-rays showed evidence of an old, healing fracture of her left femoral shaft.

◆ Diagnosis: Axis I—No Psychiatric Disorder

The initially somewhat obscure presentation of a physically abused child initially suggested an infectious etiology. A more thorough examination after an infectious etiology was not found led to the tragic discovery of trauma (Smith 2003). Although psychosomatic medicine psychiatrists may not have primary responsibility of cases such as this, multidisciplinary evaluation of the psychosocial environment of the child can lead to targeted inquiries and interventions to facilitate a safe placement for the child. Such cases often produce strong countertransference in medical center personnel, and the psychosomatic medicine psychiatrist may be of assistance in the liaison function with nursing staff and physician colleagues involved in the care of the child.

Pancreatitis and Risperidone in a Child

The patient was an 8-year-old white male with a history of oppositional, aggressive, and violent behavior with hallucinations. He was started on risperidone 0.5 mg bid with improved control of psychiatric symptoms. However, 4 weeks later, he presented with abdominal pain that was diagnosed as pancreatitis. His lipase was 292 U; his amylase was 246 U/dL. Computed tomography scan confirmed a pancreatic pseudocyst, which was drained surgically. His amylase peaked at 583 U/dL and lipase at 1,290 U before both gradually normalized. Risperidone was held. Despite the hold on antipsychotic medication, his behavior remained stable during hospitalization. After 3 weeks of hospitalization, his pancreatitis had cleared and he was discharged.

◆ **Diagnosis: Axis I—Psychotic Disorder Not Otherwise Specified, 298.9; Adverse Effects of Medication Not Otherwise Specified, 995.2**

Pancreatitis as a side effect of risperidone treatment is rare; it is likely rarer still in pediatric patients. Psychosomatic medicine physicians treating children for psychotic or delirium symptoms should be aware of this rare but very uncomfortable condition, which may require a significant period of hospitalization and supportive care.

Reference

Smith J: Shaken baby syndrome. Orthop Nurs 22:196–205, 2003

16

PAIN

The management of pain, often acute or chronic, in the medical center is associated with the need for creative use of psychopharmacology. These cases are often highly individualized and present ethical and even legal dilemmas as well. Often the psychosomatic medicine psychiatrist must assist the admitting clinical services and the pain management consultation services in creative co-management (or even "tri-management") of these patients.

Acute or Chronic Pain, Opioid Dependence, Opioid Withdrawal, and Methadone

The patient was a 44-year-old woman admitted with several fractured ribs to a community hospital after a motor vehicle accident. After several days, she developed abdominal pain and lightheadedness as well as systolic hypotension. A ruptured spleen was suspected, and she was transferred to a major medical center for splenectomy, performed without incident soon after arrival. The surgical team noted that she was taking 60 mg of methadone for long-standing opiate dependence, however, and asked for a psychiatry consult. The surgical fellow managing the case knew that the medical center did not have a license to prescribe methadone for the indication of addiction, and she summarized her fears about the situation, saying, "I don't want to lose my license for some drug addict!" Furthermore, she had prescribed nothing other than acetaminophen for postsurgical pain after the splenectomy.

The consulting psychiatrist found a somewhat uncomfortable-appearing woman who was more than happy to tell her story. Without any apparent prevarication, she admitted that she had been taking methadone for more than 10 years, since being caught stealing opioids from the hospital where she worked. A registered nurse, she used the opioids to treat her frequent migraine headaches but soon became opioid dependent. If she missed a day she would have withdrawal symptoms, and despite successful chemical-dependence treatment, she had never been able to taper off opioids. Her prescribing physician at the community facility, an internist and director of the methadone clinic, provided the collateral history that she had been a "model patient." She had never had a "dirty" urine specimen and had never abused her methadone. They both agreed that the hypertension, nausea, and body tremors she experienced with even the smallest taper in her dosage precluded her discontinuing the medication.

At this point, the surgical team refused to prescribe methadone for a patient at risk of going into serious opioid withdrawal. The consulting psychiatrist decided that emergent consultation from the medical center's legal staff was required to clarify the legal implications of the case. Despite the fears of the surgeon, the attorney's opinion was that she would be completely within bounds prescribing methadone for this patient. The attorney's reasoning was that the patient came to the hospital for a surgical emergency, not for maintenance treatment of her opioid dependence or detoxification. The methadone should be regarded as one of her ongoing medications, prescribed as any other would be, until she could return to the care of the outpatient provider licensed to treat her chronic opioid dependence in an ongoing way.

The psychiatrist recommended that the anesthesia pain management service weigh in on appropriate management of the patient's postoperative pain. The surgeon ultimately prescribed the methadone, plus additional opioids for postsurgical pain, which the pain management service recommended be tapered before the patient left the hospital. The surgeon also reviewed the situation with the community internist, who assured her of his intent to continue working with the patient for chronic treatment after her hospital discharge.

◆ **Diagnosis: Axis I—Opioid Dependence, 304.00; Opioid Withdrawal, 292.0; Pain Disorder Associated With Both Psychological Factors and a General Medical Condition, 307.89**

In the management of acute pain, particularly postoperative pain, it is necessary at times to address the acute pain management needs in ways that may superficially appear at odds with the chronic management. There is great concern generally about the use of opioids in methadone-maintenance patients, for fear of iatrogenically encouraging an exacerbation of the underlying problem of opioid dependence. Paradoxically, the administrative and legal constraints in place for methadone maintenance treatment for "typical" cases of opioid dependence may (as in this case) be seen by clinicians as administratively limiting the options for acute management of methadone-maintenance patients in the acute medical and surgical setting. The approach here, a practical one, is to "split off" the acute management (including the reasonable and appropriate short-term postsurgical use of opioids) from the longer-term management (outpatient methadone maintenance for chronic opioid dependence). As is illustrated here, close clinical coordination between the acute care team in the medical center and the eventual return to outpatient management is highly desirable for continuity of care.

Pain, Substance Dependence, and Cushing's Syndrome

Patients with endocrine illnesses may have associated behavioral correlates and complications that come to the attention of the psychosomatic medicine psychiatrist. Maintaining a sense of balance between endocrinological and behavioral problems may be a challenge to the clinicians involved in the care of these patients.

> The patient was a 36-year-old man with ongoing complications of Cushing's syndrome in the context of ectopic adrenocorticotropic hormone (ACTH) production. He had a "colorful" past that included national ranking as a wrestler during high school and college, the fathering of several children by multiple women starting in his late teens, high achievement in the trades to make money to support his many children, and cocaine and methamphetamine abuse to obviate the need for sleep so that he could maintain his high-flying lifestyle and its consequences.
>
> The patient had known for at least 2 years that he had an endocrine problem. Deeply devoted to maintaining a wrestler's physique, he had sought medical attention when he experienced generalized weakness and weight gain—particularly on his torso—that he was unable to "exercise away." Told by doctors that he had Cushing's syndrome, he redoubled his exercise regimen and did not choose to seek further treatment until he found himself frequently falling, the

result of his legs giving way beneath him from reduced muscle tone and impaired sensation. He also was experiencing occasional bouts of both urinary and rectal incontinence.

As part of his efforts to combat his burgeoning health problems, he had given up stimulants more than a year earlier. Admitted to an outside hospital with acute onset of abdominal pain, he underwent laparotomy that was inconclusive. Postoperatively, however, he developed acute, intense back pain. He had been open about his substance abuse history prior to surgery, but when he told his doctors about his back pain, they refused to give him opioids, accusing him of drug-seeking behavior.

The patient had told the doctors he had Cushing's syndrome, and they could see it. But the patient did not make the connection between his pain and the Cushing's, and neither did the doctors. His assertion, borne out by the evidence, was that the doctors refused initially to look further into his back pain because they had decided he was a drug abuser, in this case not connecting that bone pathology is a complication of Cushing's syndrome.

Discharge was planned with him still complaining of intense pain. With a social worker advocating for him after he refused to leave the hospital until his pain was managed, the surgical team finally ordered spinal films that showed multiple collapsed vertebrae, possibly sustained during his abdominal operation.

At this point, confronted with objective evidence of severe bone pathology, his doctors saw his pain in a different light. No longer were they focused on his substance abuse history, but rather they appreciated—for the first time—that he had classic stigmata of advanced Cushing's syndrome, including moon facies, limb wasting, abdominal striae, truncal obesity, osteoporosis, and yellowed skin, and that his back pain was another manifestation of his Cushing's syndrome. Transferred to a major medical center, he was judged to be in adrenal crisis and underwent emergent bilateral adrenalectomy. He was found to have extensive lymphomatosis of his lower spinal column, which explained his gait difficulties and incontinence. He ultimately required laminectomies of multiple vertebral bodies for osteoporotic changes. These changes had set the stage for the spinal stress fractures that became symptomatic after surgery. After an extensive workup, an ACTH-producing tumor was identified in the apex of his left lung. He underwent thoracotomy to remove the tumor and eventually had surgery to repair multiple abdominal hernias, the result of poor wound healing in his hypercortisolemic state.

◆ **Diagnosis: Axis I—Opioid Abuse, 305.50; Amphetamine Abuse, 305.70; Axis II—Rule Out Narcissistic Personality Disorder, 301.81**

Patients with character pathology, especially when associated with substance abuse, may cause significant countertransference reactions in medical providers. These patients' behaviors may lead to accusations of "noncompliance" and "drug-seeking" and may obscure systemic illnesses underlying their clinical problems (such as severe pain in this case). Despite the fact that this man was told early in the course of his illness about his Cushing's syndrome, his attempts to "exercise" away his physical stigmata may have represented either a maladaptive denial of illness or, at the very least, a maladaptive coping with his illness. Once he became significantly systemically ill with many complications, his case could be seen in a different light.

17

PSYCHOSIS IN THE GENERAL MEDICAL SETTING

Finally, we share cases in which psychosis, although outside the context of delirium or dementia, nonetheless presents in a particularly disruptive manner in the general medical setting.

The King of the Leprechauns, "Beware of the Nazis!" and "The Eagle Has Landed"

Occasionally the clinician will encounter fascinating delusional patients on the inpatient medical and surgical wards. Although these individuals are really best thought of as chronic psychotic disorder patients with incidental need for medical and surgical hospitalization, their psychotic symptoms, when shared, will be seen as extreme to the admitting medical and surgical teams. Sometimes (as in the cases that follow) and somewhat remarkably, these patients will have somehow avoided mental health treatment despite what appear to be extremely disabling psychotic symptoms, including remarkably elaborate delusional belief systems. Once their acute medical and surgical issues are managed, these patients may need involuntary commitment to a psychiatric facility for their chronic psychotic disorders. Although these cases are not truly "psychosomatic" in nature, they are encountered in a psychosomatic context and tend to be memorable to the medical and surgical units.

> The first patient was a 60-year-old single white male who was admitted to the general medicine service for management of chronic obstructive pulmonary disorder. He had a relatively uncomplicated

course medically and recovered well with conservative treatment. However, his behavior and delusions were (to a medicine service) extremely disruptive. This man claimed to be "500 years old." He also claimed to have lived all over the world, "but mostly in Ireland and Scotland." Despite not having an ethnically Celtic name, he spoke in an Irish accent. This was, he claimed, because of his "special position in Ireland and Scotland as the 'King of the Leprechauns.'" He believed he had had this title bestowed on him "in the Middle Ages," and by now, several hundred years later, he had charge of a large group of (subordinate) leprechauns "all over the world" who worked for him. He explained, in a calm and matter-of-fact way, that the reason he had been chosen as the "King" was because as a normal-sized man (he was of average height), he was so much larger than the "other" leprechauns that he was the logical choice to be the one in charge. When asked what color was the skin of leprechauns, he said that "the other leprechauns" were green but that he had "white skin because I am not only a large leprechaun, I am an albino, too." This allowed him to more easily live in society where his "leprechaun" identity could be concealed. He had no close family members, was not employed, and could not describe a safe plan of self-care. Because of his inability to describe a self-care plan and his elaborate delusions, he was committed to an inpatient psychiatric facility for further evaluation and treatment.

◆ Diagnosis: Axis I—Schizophrenia, Undifferentiated Type, 295.90

The second patient was a 29-year-old single white male. He was admitted to the trauma service after being struck by a light rail train and with a blood alcohol level of greater than 400 mg/dL. Fortunately, his injuries were managed without complications and he had a good prognosis for physical recovery. Upon psychosomatic medicine interview he revealed, in addition to his daily heavy alcohol consumption, an elaborate delusional belief system. He was walking on the light rail tracks, he explained, on a critical mission to save the Earth. Only if he balanced himself while walking on the train rail could the "universe stay on track." He feared that if he had fallen off of the rail the "Universe would have disintegrated—that's why I didn't get off when I saw the train coming." Furthermore, he explained, the universe is threatened "because the U.S. soldiers have secretly been replaced by a bunch of Nazis" and were, as a result, untrustworthy. He then produced an elaborate notebook with what appeared to be a pictorial code. The message in his little book, he claimed, contained all the "background information" about the

"Nazi plot to take over the government." He had not brought the book or his concerns to the attention to any government figures "because I am afraid that the one I speak to will be in on the conspiracy too." Remarkably, he had not been previously identified as needing mental health treatment, despite apparently several years of clearly and floridly delusional thinking about these paranoid themes. After he was no longer in need of inpatient trauma care, he was sent to the psychiatric inpatient facility for further evaluation and care.

◆ **Diagnosis: Axis I—Schizophrenia, Paranoid Type, 295.30**

The third patient was a 35-year-old white male with a history of substance dependence who had developed a movement disorder. Although he had abused stimulants, hallucinogens, and other drugs over the years, it was never definitively established whether his movement disorder (consisting of parkinsonian symptoms) was a direct consequence of his substance abuse. He was admitted for evaluation of his movement disorder. Psychosomatic medicine consultation was ordered to "evaluate delusions."

Upon interview, he explained that he had been "transformed" into the "spirit of an eagle." This was the result of a revelatory experience that may have followed drug intoxication. He claimed that having "become an eagle" gave him "the powers of flight" and the "ability to understand enlightenment." He began flapping his upper extremities in an attempt to "actually fly," which was alarming to the staff because he had been admitted to one of the upper floors of the hospital. A 24-hour sitter was assigned to him because of concerns that he might actually try to fly out of the window in response to his delusions. He was treated with quetiapine and within several days announced to the psychosomatic medicine team "I am now fully lucid, I am no longer delusional, and I am no longer an eagle."

◆ **Diagnosis: Axis I—Psychotic Disorder Not Otherwise Specified, 298.9; Other Substance Dependence, 304.90**

These three patients, all with classic, if remarkably elaborate, delusional belief systems, were identified for treatment as a result of psychosomatic medicine consultation. Such patients may be seen as variably amusing, perplexing, and sometimes frightening to the medical and surgical wards that we serve. Given these patients' chronic illness, it is unclear how much they might improve in the short term, even with intensive inpatient mental health treatment.

It was remarkable in these cases that such delusional and nearly disorganized patients had somehow managed to avoid mental health evaluation until seen for evaluation in a psychosomatic medicine context. In the third case, the delusional symptoms resolved after quetiapine was started; whether this man had a chronic or intermittent illness connected to his movement disorder or substance abuse remained speculative. This patient's safety had to be assured in the event that he actually attempted to fly while in the delusional stance that he was an eagle. Psychosomatic medicine psychiatrists should remain vigilant for the occasional, dramatic, and quite memorable chronically delusional patient encountered in the medical and surgical services.

Hallucinated Animals, Real Weapon

The patient was a 65-year-old white male with a history of mild dementia. He was seen in consultation because of his acting-out behavior. He had for some time been "seeing animals" in his home. They were described as "small and furry" and "all over the house." These "animals" were not seen by anyone else in his home. After tolerating the hallucinated animals and becoming frustrated that his family members could not also "see" them, the patient took matters into his own hands. He loaded his shotgun and proceeded to shoot at the hallucinated animals. His family, obviously disrupted by the live gunfire in the house, managed to persuade him to surrender the weapon and to seek out a clinical evaluation.

Examination revealed mild cognitive impairment with no suicidal or homicidal ideations. He did not complain of "animals" in his hospital room but was very insistent in his account that there "really were" animals in his home. The lack of actual animals in the home was confirmed by several family members. He was prescribed a low dose of risperidone, with the most important clinical intervention being the complete removal of all weapons from the home.

◆ **Diagnosis: Axis I—Dementia Not Otherwise Specified, 294.8**

A point that is obvious to the practicing clinician is the toxic combination of access to weapons and cognitive impairment. The patient's visual hallucinations, which were nonbizarre and very convincing, only came to clinical attention when he shot at the hallucinations. It is likely that hallucinations of animals may be more likely to provoke this sort of response because, to some degree, shooting at intruding animals is an act that has at least some social support. As such, the act of shooting at "animals" believed to be there is not considered to be as "disinhibited" an act as it would if the patient, for example, had shot at another human whom he experienced as threatening. Nonetheless, the access to lethal means in a cognitively impaired patient is very dangerous indeed. The first clinical intervention of disarming this man was far more urgent than the psychopharmacological treatment of his hallucinations.

DIAGNOSIS INDEX

DSM-IV-TR® diagnoses and diagnostic codes grouped by DSM category. Page numbers printed in **boldface** type refer to tables.

Disorders Usually Diagnosed in Infancy, Childhood, or Adolescence

299.80   Asperger's disorder
      rule out, 243–246, **247**, 248
314.00   Attention-deficit/hyperactivity disorder, predominantly inattentive type, 148–150
314.9   Attention-deficit/hyperactivity disorder not otherwise specified, 199–202
317   Mild mental retardation, 199–202

Delirium, Dementia, and Amnestic and Other Cognitive Disorders

294.0   Amnestic disorder due to carbon monoxide poisoning, 60–62
294.9   Cognitive disorder not otherwise specified, 229–231, 265–266, 266–267
      due to acute effects of electroconvulsive therapy (presumed), 22–24
      rule out, 243–246, **247**, 248
293.0   Delirium, 7–8, 12–13, 20–21, 25–27, 27–28, 28–29, 28–30, 28–31, 31–32, 33, 38–41, 41–43, 45–48, 48–50, 62–63, 71–72, 76–78, 86–87, 98–100, 100–103, 131–134, 138–142, 143–146, 164–168, 172–176, 185–189, 192–194, 194–196, 196–197, 209–212, 221–224, 227–229, 231–233, 261–263, 263–264
      due to interleukin-2, 146–148
      due to liver disease, 78–80
      in remission, 219–221
      resolved, 95–98
294.10   Dementia of the Alzheimer's type, 275–277, 276–277
294.11   Dementia of the Alzheimer's type, with behavioral disturbance, 248–251
294.10   Dementia due to a general medical condition, 267–268
294.11   Dementia due to a general medical condition, with behavioral disturbance, 225–227, 259–260
      due to the fragile X tremor/ataxia syndrome, 255–258
294.8   Dementia not otherwise specified, 292–293
      rule out, 227–229
290.42   Vascular dementia, with delusions, 271–272
290.43   Vascular dementia, with depressed mood, 45–48, 98–100
      rule out, 268–271

SUBJECT INDEX

Page numbers printed in **boldface** type refer to tables.

"Triple D triangle"
(dementia, delirium, depression),
45–46, 47–48
Trust, 69
TTE. *See* Transthoracic
echocardiogram

Uterine cancer, 138–142

Valium (diazepam), 210–211
Valproate, 78
delirium with, 25–28
Valproic acid
for treatment of delirium
and/or agitation, 28–33
for treatment of manic
episodes, 95
Vancomycin, 168
Vascular dementia, 45–48, 98–100,
271–272

Venlafaxine, 255
for treatment of delirium, 27
for treatment of depression, 82,
83–84, 213, 258
Viral encephalitis, malignant catatonia
and, 164–168
Visual impairment, 11–13

Warfarin, 131
Wilson disease, 225–227
Wounds
diabetes mellitus and, 68
self-inflicted puncture wounds
to the eyes, 197–198
self-inflicted stab wound to the
heart, 55–56

Ziprasidone, 41, 49, 78
Zolpidem, 76, 151, 172, 227